Badass Body Goals:
The Booty Shaping &
Resistance Training Journal

Created with love by
Jennifer Cohen, Amir Atighehchi, Ariel Banayan, & Mikey Ahdoot

Copyright ©2019 Every Damn Day, LLC

All rights reserved.

Published by Every Damn Day, LLC.

No part of this publication may be reproduced, or stored in a retrieval system, or transmitted in any form or by any means, electronic, mechanical, recording, photocopying, scanning or otherwise, without express written permission of the publisher.

For information about permission to reproduce elections from this book, email team@habitnest.com

Visit our website at www.HabitNest.com

PUBLISHER'S DISCLAIMER

While the publisher and author have used their best efforts in preparing this book, they make no representations or warranties with respect to the accuracy or completeness of the contents of this book. The advice and strategies contained herein may not be suitable for your situation. You should consult with a professional where appropriate. Neither the publisher nor the author shall be liable for any loss of profit or any other commercial damages, including but not limited to special, incidental, consequential, or other damages.

The company, product, and service names used in this book are for identification purposes only. All trademarks and registered trademarks are the property of their respective owners.

ISBN: 9780998656175

SECOND EDITION

Exercises Disclaimer:

The exercises provided by Habit Nest™ & Jennifer Cohen (and habitnest.com) are for educational and entertainment purposes only, and is not to be interpreted as a recommendation for a specific treatment plan, product, or course of action. Exercise is not without its risks, and this or any other exercise program may result in injury. They include but are not limited to: risk of injury, aggravation of a pre-existing condition, or adverse effect of over-exertion such as muscle strain, abnormal blood pressure, fainting, disorders of heartbeat, and very rare instances of heart attack. To reduce the risk of injury, before beginning this or any exercise program, please consult a healthcare provider for appropriate exercise prescription and safety precautions. The exercise instruction and advice presented are in no way intended as a substitute for medical consultation. Habit Nest™ disclaims any liability from and in connection with this program. As with any exercise program, if at any point during your workout you begin to feel faint, dizzy, or have physical discomfort, you should stop immediately and consult a physician.

Information Disclaimer:

The information provided by Habit Nest™ (and habitnest.com) is for educational and entertainment purposes only, and is not to be interpreted as a recommendation for a specific treatment plan. Habit Nest™ does not provide specific medical advice, and is not engaged in providing medical services. Habit Nest ™ does not replace consultation with a qualified health or medical professional who sees you in person, for the health and medical needs of yourself or a loved one. In addition, while Habit Nest ™ frequently updates contents, medical, health and fitness information changes rapidly, and therefore, some information may be out of date. Please see a physician or health professional immediately if you suspect you may be ill or injured.

Table of Contents

1 The Unvarnished Truth
- *Which Booty Shape Do YOU Have?*
- *A Little Booty-ology*

4 How We're Going To Get You The Best Butt Ever
- *Top Reasons People Have Trouble Shaping Their Butts*
- *Testing For A Glute Imbalance*
- *Glute Activation*
- *'Angling'*
- *Building A Strong Core*

10 How The Journal Works
- *4-3-2-1 Workouts*
- *Weight Training*

19 Some Fat Loss Science
- *Achieving A Caloric Deficit*
- *Carbohydrates, Proteins, & Fats*
- *Taking Action On Your Nutrition Goals*

35 Goal-Setting Principles
- *Perfectionists, Tread Lightly*
- *Developing Strength From The Inside Out*
- *You Are Perfect As You Are*
- *Commit*

43 Workouts 1 - 10 + Check-In
63 Workouts 11 - 20 + Check-In
83 Workouts 21 - 30 + Check-In
103 Workouts 31 - 40 + Check-In
123 Workouts 41 - 50 + Finished!

144 Fin

The Unvarnished Truth

Whether you have a naturally athletic build, a figure that's curvaceous, or one that's willowy, there's good news:

You can develop most of the physical attributes you've always wanted but didn't get from Mother Nature or your gene pool.

The truth is, with strategic work, anyone can become fitter, stronger, more toned, more self-assured, and sexier.

That's an outcome that's realistic and healthy — for anybody.

With the right physical and psychological moves, you can turn the body you have into the body you want - losing inches, dropping pounds, and developing a stronger, more sculpted look and greater mental fortitude in the process.

If the goal of getting fit, shaping your lower body, and trimming your waist has seemed too daunting in the past, you were probably going about achieving it in the wrong way.

Sorry to lay that on you, but it's *the unvarnished truth*.

Maximizing your fitness potential isn't as difficult or taxing as many people make it out to be.

It involves four critical elements:

1. A blend of strength-training workouts,
2. The right type of cardiovascular exercise, and
3. Targeting your muscles at different angles to achieve the exact look you want.
4. Consistency.

Combine these cornerstones of fitness with healthy eating habits - upgrading the nutritional quality of your food choices by using food primarily as fuel, eating regularly, snacking strategically, and you'll soon be on your way to a leaner, stronger, fitter physique with a chiseled waist line and tight tush.

Which Booty Shape Do YOU Have?

The reality is that we each come in different beautiful shapes and sizes. Our booties look different based on our skeletal structure and the amount of muscle and fat on our differing bodies. But no matter the shape of your skeleton, you can change the way your butt looks through diet and the right type of exercise.

Think of it like this - someone who is 4'11 obviously has different possibilities for the way they're body can look than someone who is 5'11. But, both of these people still have the potential to transform their bodies in ways that maximize their body potential.

The Four Main Shapes Of The Derrière:

Although you should be able to pick out which type of booty you have from these pictures, even if there isn't an *exact* match, these are only meant as a guide. We're all too different to have exact categories we each fit into!

HEART/PEAR ('A' SHAPE)   INVERTED ('V' SHAPE)   ROUND ('O' SHAPE)   SQUARE ("H" SHAPE)

The Heart/Pear Shape ('A'): This type of butt results from fat distribution around the lower portion of the butt and thighs, leading to an increase in widening from the waist down to the `bottom of the butt. Underdeveloped heart/pear shaped butts are commonly referred to as 'Saddlebags'.

The Inverted 'V' Shape: The 'V' shape becomes more common as we age because lower estrogen levels change the place of fat storage from the butt to the midsection. It gives the look of the bottom of the butt being less full than the top, resulting in a 'V' shape.

The Round 'O' Shape: Also known as 'the bubble butt', this type of booty is the result of fat distribution around the whole butt cheek.

The Square 'H' Shape: This shape is the result of prominent hip bones (the structure of the pelvis) and distribution of fat in the hips (also known as love handles), giving the more vertical look on the sides of the glutes.

No matter which type of booty you do have, we're going to make sure to get you the booty shape you *want* to have.

A Little Booty-ology

Let's take just a moment to talk about about your derrière.

It's really important to understand a little bit about how vital butt health is to the functioning of your body, and get familiar with the different parts of the booty that need to be developed for the best overall shape and size.

Your butt is made of pure muscle, and is probably the most important muscle in your entire body.

But your booty isn't just one muscle - it's a combination of three primary muscles groups called:

The Gluteus Maximus: The biggest muscle in the area, responsible for extending the leg backwards and rotating the pelvis and thighs.

The Gluteus Medius: Located on top of the gluteus maximus that raises the log out and to the side while promoting overall body-balance.

The Gluteus Minimus: Residing under the upper part of the gluteus maximus, and works with the gluteus medius.

Although the Gluteus Maximus is the largest muscle in the area, all three muscle groups are important to both your every day functioning, and the shape of your butt.

Strong glutes help support the core, decrease your risk of serious injury, improve posture, and of course, help your butt look great in any outfit.

Regardless of your genetics, you can shape your butt any way you want if you understand the different shapes your booty can take and create a plan of action that will steer you towards your goal.

In the next section, we'll discuss why so many people find it difficult, and help you understand exactly how we're going to get you the look you want.

How We're Going To Get You The Best Butt Ever

The TOP reasons people have trouble lifting, shaping, and toning their butts:

1. Not 'activating' the glute muscles (not firing the glute muscles)
2. Muscle imbalances
3. Training methods that don't work
4. Repeating the same movements over and over again
5. Not enough weight training
6. Over-training the gluteus maximus and under training the gluteus medius, gluteus minimis, hamstrings, and adductor muscles
7. Not eating well enough
8. Not training consistently enough
9. Incorrect technique and form, causing compensation with the other muscle groups such as the quadriceps

Failing to activate the glute muscles and instead overcompensating by using other parts of the body to do the exercises you're performing is the easiest way to delay your progress and potentially injure yourself.

The second biggest problem leading to a lack of results is not targeting each part of the glute muscles with a variety of exercises to hit the butt muscles at every possible angle.

Testing For A Glute Imbalance

Glute imbalances lead to a failure to activate the glute muscles.

Glute imbalances are very common because of the simple fact that our sedentary lifestyles cause our butts to become 'dormant' over time.

Consistently sitting for long periods of time causes the hip flexors to tighten and the glute muscles to weaken, leading to decreased strength and stabilization in our butts.

This decreased strength and activation of the glute muscles leads to muscle imbalances and an assortment of injuries to our lower backs and legs.

Some Words Like "Butt"

- Rear End
- Hind End
- Hiney
- Glutes
- Posterior
- Rear
- Can
- Cheeks
- Derrière
- Fanny
- Bum
- Butt
- Behind
- Ass
- Arse

Here are some exercises to determine whether you have a glute imbalance, or difficulty activating or firing your glute muscles:

1. Stand on one foot with one leg lifted for one minute. Then do the same thing with the other leg.

2. Get into a table-top position with your hands directly underneath your shoulders. From here, pull your abs in towards your spine so your back is straight, and extend one leg up while contracting the glute muscles in that leg as tightly as possible. Then, perform the same movement with the other leg.

3. Air Squats: Standing up, separate your feet so that they're shoulder-width apart. Keeping your back straight and your toes pointed straight forward, bend your knees so that your butt goes down towards the floor. As you perform the movement, make sure your knees are moving straight up and down rather than bending forward past your toes. Complete the movement repeatedly until it burns too much to do anymore. When it gets difficult, pay attention to whether you lean to one side of your body as you complete the movement.

After performing these exercises, answer the following questions:

1. In the first exercise, was there one leg you felt more stable on at the end of the minute?

2. When completing the exercises above, do you feel contraction in your glute muscles or does it feel like your hamstrings and/or quadriceps are doing all of the work?

3. When performing the first two exercises, did you have an easier time contracting one side as compared to the other?

4. Do you feel that your glute muscles on one side are bigger or stronger than the other side?

5. When performing the air squat exercise, did you favor one side of your body over the other by leaning in that direction?

If your answer to any of the above questions is 'yes', chances are you have some level of a glute imbalance and/or difficulty activating your glute muscles. Without correcting glute imbalances and making sure you're *activating* the glute muscles, your legs and booty cannot transform into the shape you want because the right muscles aren't being properly trained. Imbalanced or uneven glutes won't just affect the quality of your results, but they'll impact ability to properly and safely perform pretty much any lower body exercise! Our program combats the issues that arise from glute imbalances by specifically taking steps to ensure your glutes are 'activating' properly as you perform each exercise.

Now, let's talk about 'Glute Activation'

The harsh reality is that most people don't actually activate the muscles in their butts when doing their workout routine.

When someone really understands the importance of glute activation, it adds a whole new quality to their tushy workouts.

Glute activation is just a fancy phrase to represent the idea that the muscles in your butt should be working or 'firing' properly when you perform exercises intended to target those muscles.

Activating the glute muscles is like waking them up from a deep sleep so that they're ready for the workout. It's just like drinking coffee in the morning, except for your butt!

Important Steps For Getting Your Glute Muscles Firing:

1. Building the mind-muscle connection

When you want to do any physical movement, your brain releases a neurotransmitter called **acetylcholine** that stimulates the muscles to move.

What's remarkable is that research has found that the more active attention you place on the muscle you want to move, the more acetylcholine the brain releases.

In other words, the more mental attention you give to your butt muscles as you're performing each repetition of an exercise, the better the muscle contracts and 'fires.'

So, bringing your mind into your booty as you workout is crucial!

2. Loosening up your tight butt muscles and making sure they're firing

You loosen your butt muscles and activate them by completing simple movements that allow you to really *feel* the glute muscles contracting so you can aim to feel the same contraction throughout each exercise.

We're going to begin each workout with a **resistance-band warmup** to wake your booty up so your entire lower body is primed for the best possible results.

The good news: Because the glutes are the biggest muscle in your body, they have the most room for change. The results will come quickly if you put in the work!

Angling

One of the problems many people have with training their butts stems from thinking of their butt as one muscle.

In reality, the butt is made up of a group of different muscles that each require unique movements from every direction to target the different parts for the overall best possible shape.

You need to make sure to target and develop each muscle that makes up your butt.

By incorporating unique variations of each exercise,
we'll make sure that you're targeting each key part of the butt and leg muscles consistently so that your entire lower body is being developed for the best possible results.

Building A Strong Core

If you really want to develop a strong core - which is an essential part of almost every physical movement you make throughout the course of your day - you need to challenge all the muscles in the abdomen.

- *The rectus abdominis* (the two bands of muscle that run down the center of your abdomen),
- *The transverse abdominis* (the muscle that wraps horizontally around your lower abdomen), and
- *The internal and external obliques* (which form the innermost and outermost layers that run down the sides of your waist).
- *The Mid & Lower Back*

In other words, to build true core strength you need to work the muscles that are deep inside your core, not just the superficial muscles.

Building a strong core is important for lots of reasons.

For starters, the muscles in your core (your whole torso) provide the girdle or corset that supports your entire body.

Developing a powerful core can reduce your risk of experiencing lower back pain or other injury.

By contrast, neglecting these crucial muscles can shortchange you of the stability your body needs for a variety of movements in daily life.

Having a weak core is like turning off your body's power center and trying to rely only on satellite forms of energy instead (by compensating for physical movement with other muscles that the core should be the primary factor in).

Keep in mind though, that if ripped abs are your goal, no amount of core training guarantees you'll get them.

Abs aren't necessarily 'made' in the kitchen - the muscles themselves are developed in the gym. BUT, without working just as hard in the kitchen as you do in the gym, your abs won't ever show the way you want them to!

How Often Should I Exercise?

This is a common question that is situational based on what's realistic for each person.

The journal is structured to be undated and used by what works for you, your goals, and your schedule.

As a frame of reference:

- **Light**: Exercise 2 days a week.

- **Medium**: Exercise 4 days a week.

- **Hard**: Exercise 5-6 days a week.

If you're driven enough to achieve the best results, you should set a long-term goal of building up to 5-6 workouts a week.

How The Journal Works

Every day, you're going to be given a complete workout routine consisting of:

1. How long the workout will take
2. Exactly which exercises to perform
3. Images showing how to perform each exercise
4. The duration of each exercise
5. The optimal duration for your resting periods

Your have two tasks to complete on days you choose to workout:

1. <u>Before you get to the gym (or right before you start)</u>:
   Look at what the day's workout consists of - which exercises you'll be doing - and read the explanations in the workout index in the back of the journal. Alternatively, you can visit the "Exercise Guide" link listed on each page which contain video walkthroughs of how to complete each exercise for that day.

Until you're familiar with each exercise, it'll be annoying to keep looking back at the index during your workout so it would be wise to get familiar with the exercises the night before or for 5 minutes before you begin.

2. <u>During your workout</u>: Fill in the amount of repetitions you did for each exercise. You could either do this quickly after each exercise, after each set, or during the 30s break following each circuit.

We designate tracking lines for all of this, you just have to write down the numbers. This is one of the ways you'll be tracking your progress to see how far along you've come!

You can see the flow of a sample workout on the next page.

Sample 4-3-2-1 Workout

Three of the *five* workouts for the week will be what we call the '4-3-2-1' method. *Each of the workouts will have a warmup followed by four circuits, broken down as followed*:

Begin 3-5min Warmup

 GLUTE ACTIVATION WARMUP

a. Clam Opener   **b. Glute Bridge w/ Band Flutter**   **c. Tabletop w/ Donkey Kick**   **d. Lateral Leg Raise**

(30s Each Side)   (30s Each Side)   - 30s Each Leg (w/ Foot Flexed)
                                                                                                                                                        - 30s Each Leg (w/ Toes Pointing Down)

Begin "4-3-2-1" Workout

<u>Circuit 1:</u> Perform these four exercises for 60 seconds each.
(*You'll do this entire circuit once* with no break in between exercises).

 CIRCUIT 1

1a. High Knee   **1b. Bulgarian Lunge**   **1c. Bulgarian Lunge**   **1d. Side V-Up**

  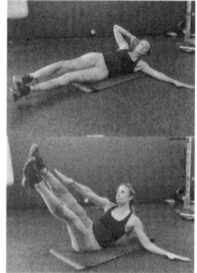

REPS: _____ → REPS: _____ → REPS: _____ → REPS: _____
                             (Right Leg)   (Left Leg)   (30s Each Side)

Now, take your first break for 30 seconds.

Circuit 2: Perform these three exercises for 50 seconds each.
*(You'll do this entire circuit **twice** with no break in between any exercises or sets).*

 CIRCUIT 2
50s EACH

2a. Side Shuffle w/ Floor Tap

2b. Plank Step Up

2c. In and Out Jack

SET 1 REPS: _____   →   SET 1 REPS: _____   →   SET 1 REPS: _____

SET 2 REPS: _____   →   SET 2 REPS: _____   →   SET 2 REPS: _____

Now, take your second break for 30 seconds.

Circuit 3: Perform these two exercises for 40 seconds each.
*(You'll do this circuit **three times** with no break in between any exercises or sets).*

CIRCUIT 3
40s EACH

3a. Side Plank w/ Torso Twist

3b. Lateral Lunge w/ Half 'X'

(Left Side)   SET 1 REPS: _____   →   (Left Side)   SET 1 REPS: _____

(Right Side)   SET 2 REPS: _____   →   (Right Side)   SET 2 REPS: _____

(Alternate Side)   SET 3 REPS: _____   →   (Alternate Side)   SET 3 REPS: _____

Now, take your third break for 30 seconds.

Circuit 4: Perform this one exercise for 30 seconds.
(You'll do this circuit **four times** with a **15 second break** in between each set).

 CIRCUIT 4

4a. Pendulum Jack

SET 1 REPS: _____ → 15s REST
SET 2 REPS: _____ → 15s REST
SET 3 REPS: _____ → 15s REST
SET 4 REPS: _____ → 15s REST

Now, take your fourth break for 30 seconds.

Begin Cool Down

COOL DOWN — 60s EACH

a. Hamstring Stretch   **b. Runner's Stretch**   **c. Butterfly Stretch**   **d. Lat Stretch**

Done!

Note: we created a video timer specifically to guide you through your 4-3-2-1 workouts (especially when beginning) to help you get the hang of it. You can view these on the top left of each workout.

EXERCISE GUIDE — HabitNest.link/booty01

Each workout follows a 4-3-2-1 pattern; the specific exercises for each are described in detail in the workout index in the back of the book or via the Exercise Video Guide links listed on each workout page.

The four circuits in the actual workout will take you about 25 minutes to complete, including the warmup, cool-down, and **30-second break after each circuit**.

One day per week, the entire 4-3-2-1 workout will be dedicated to sculpting your butt and legs.

A second day of it will primarily aim to trim your waist line and developing your core and abdominal muscles.

A third day of it will have an ideal mix of lower body and upper body exercises for well-rounded muscle development and toning.

Why Use The '4-3-2-1' Method?

The 4-3-2-1 method is fundamentally rooted in *High Intensity Interval Training (HIIT)* which has been proven to torch the most fat as efficiently as possible.

Getting stronger and fitter is really a two-step process:

1. You need to do the strength training to build lean muscle mass, and
2. You need to do the right forms of cardiovascular exercise to burn body fat.

This dynamic duo will deliver the strong, badass-body you want faster than any other approach (assuming you also stick with a healthy, protein-rich eating plan).

The good news is that the cardio part of the equation doesn't have to take over your life.

A 25 minute calorie-torching HIIT routine is the equivalent of 75 minutes of steady-paced cardio.

Who wouldn't want to save time and crush their fitness goals all at once?

The HIIT cardio approach embedded in the 4-3-2-1 method carries a whole bunch of specific health benefits like:

- It's the easiest way to lose belly fat while maintaining muscle mass
- Burn 3 times more calories than traditional cardiovascular workouts

- The 'After-Burn' effect causes your body to burn more calories for hours after your workout
- Chisels out your waist line
- Lowers fasting insulin and increases insulin sensitivity
- Boosts metabolism
- Improves HDL (the 'good' cholesterol)
- Reduces blood pressure
- Improves blood levels of health-protecting antioxidants

By alternating short bouts of high-intensity exercise with recovery intervals, HIIT gives you a huge bang for your buck, and it can be a fun change of pace from what you're currently accustomed to.

The main benefit of HIIT cardio over traditional cardio routines is *"the after-burn effect"* (Excess Post Exercise Oxygen Consumption):

After any ordinary, steady-state cardio routine, your body takes about two hours to restore itself to pre-exercise levels, thus using more energy and burning excess calories for a few hours after your workout.

Because of the vigorous nature of HIIT workouts, the post workout recovery demand on your body is greater and lasts longer. So, you naturally burn 15% more calories AFTER your workout than you would with an ordinary cardio routine.

In this way, we'll speed up the chiseling of your waist line by more quickly getting rid of the layer of fat around your belly.

Also, because of the nature of High Intensity Interval Training, you're targeting FAT loss rather than just losing calories.

Even more importantly, we'll be working towards building lean muscle mass *while* torching fat.

Weight Training

The two remaining workouts in the week will consist of a variety of weight training exercises to ensure that you're achieving the right muscle development to look as strong, fit, and sexy as possible!

We'll provide the exact exercises you should complete, the number of sets to do, and the number of reps to aim for.

Your job is to fill in the amount of weight you use and number of reps you actually completed in the designated tracking lines.

Why Weight Training Is Important

1. It is the most effective way to build lean muscle

For your tushy to transform into your optimal shape, you have to develop your glute muscles from all angles.

Simply put, weight-training causes the muscles to grow more quickly than other types of exercise because of the added resistance.

2. The more lean muscle mass you have, the more calories you burn naturally throughout the day, leading to faster, better results.

Your 'Basal Metabolic Rate' (**BMR**) is the number of calories you burn naturally throughout the day without exercise. This number is subject to fluctuation depending on a variety of factors. One of the big determining factors of your BMR is the amount of lean muscle mass you have. The more lean muscle mass in your body, the higher the rate at which it burns calories naturally!

3. A big component of looking 'fit' is having the right proportion and symmetry of the upper half of your body in relation to the lower half of your body.

When your upper back and shoulders are strong and toned, your waist automatically looks smaller, giving you what fitness enthusiasts call the "V" shape—otherwise known as *The V-Line Taper*.

Each exercise in this program was deliberately chosen to give you this exact look.

NOTE: *For the two rest days during the week, feel free to choose how to use them! You can take the whole weekend off or just take breaks throughout the week as needed.*

The Two Primary Factors That Determine Your Progress

The truth of the matter is that trimming your waist, shaping your butt, and burning the necessary fat for your body to look great boils down to ***two factors:***

1. Your diet
2. Doing the right type of exercise

We have you 100% covered when it comes to the proper exercise routine.

However, the effort and attention you give your diet needs to be your primary focus if you want to see the best results as quickly as possible.

Your diet provides the foundation for almost everything your body does, and it's central to any healthy fitness program.

Plus, what you eat provides the fuel for your workouts and the soothing salve for your body's post-exercise recovery. Using nutritious foods as sources of fuel, energy, and vitality will help you build lean, sculpted muscle; a healthy, resilient physique; and an overall badass body.

Some Basic Fat Loss Science

Note: Before following any nutrition advice in this journal, we recommend reaching out to your doctor and/or nutritionist to get their thoughts. This is because different people have different needs and it's always a good idea to check yours.

Achieving a Caloric Deficit

It's simple.

Your body needs a certain amount of energy to function.

A *calorie* is a unit of energy – it is the energy value of food.

When your body uses more calories than you're eating, it is forced to turn to other places to supply and fulfill the energy requirements it isn't getting from the food you're eating.

But the body has a few options for where it can go to take the energy that it needs. It can either go to fat stores, muscle protein, or a combination of both.

Our goal is to cause the body to use fat as its primary energy source.

When there is a caloric deficit and the body is forced to turn to alternate sources of energy, it is imperative to ensure that muscle catabolism doesn't occur.

Muscle catabolism is where your body uses muscle tissue for energy that it's not getting from the food you're eating.

To put everything into perspective, the moment you have a caloric surplus (you eat more calories than you burn), extra calories are stored as fat for future energy in the event that the body needs the energy later on.

Macronutrient Ratios

To lose weight, you need to eat less calories than you burn. But to cause the body to specifically burn fat, you need to **understand how the macronutrients you eat affect your body**.

The term **macronutrient** refers to the main types of food – carbohydrates, lipids (fats), and proteins.

The macronutrient ratio refers to the percentage of your caloric intake of each of these three types of foods. How much you're eating from the different food groups.

To attain the right balance that will force your body to use fat for energy while retaining muscle, your macronutrient intake has to be carefully plotted and it must be tailored to your specific body type, the speed of your metabolism, and your ordinary activity levels.

Summary:

1. Your body needs energy to function, and is in a constant state of energy expenditure.
2. A calorie is a unit of stored energy; a measure of the value of food.
3. You can force your body to burn fat by achieving a caloric deficit.
4. A caloric deficit results where you burn more calories than you consume.
5. A caloric deficit may result in your body using muscle tissue for energy, which we can prevent with a proper balance of macronutrients.

<u>Carbohydrates</u>

<u>A Double Edged Sword</u>

We need energy to live. We need energy to breathe, to digest, to circulate blood flow, to move our limbs, to think, etc. From the moment we're born until the moment we leave this beautiful world, we are using energy to facilitate our every physical movement, thought, emotion and instinctive process.

Fat loss is really about re-directing the source of that energy by manipulating the body through the foods we eat.

The body is extremely efficient. We have a very specific process for the way we create energy based on the food we eat. When there's an excess of what is needed, the body stores it to be used in a later day.

By the same token, when there's not enough energy supply, the body adapts and finds other sources.

Carbohydrates are the body's preferred source of energy.

Carbohydrates are vital to the functioning of our bodily systems. Carbs are broken down into glucose in the body. *Glucose* is the primary molecule that serves as energy for animals like us.

The main objective in achieving fat loss is forcing your body to react to circumstances you create by ***using fat for energy rather than carbohydrates or muscle*** tissue. We want our bodies to metabolize the fat that has been stored.

That happens when you don't have enough carbohydrates in your system to supply all of your energy needs, so your body releases a hormone called **glucagon**, whose job is to convert existing fat that has been stored in the body into energy the body can use.

Glycogen refers to carbs that have been stored in the body. If you're continually eating carbs, which is the favored energy source, your body has absolutely no reason to metabolize fat for energy!

What's more is that when you eat more carbs than your body needs, the excess carbohydrates that can't currently be used as energy **are stored as fat** so that they can potentially be used down the line if it becomes necessary.

A big part of fat loss is about regulating your carbohydrate intake to cause this bodily reaction of using fat as a source of energy.

But eliminating carbs completely is the wrong way to approach the task. Although it will help you achieve weight loss, you need to make sure your body isn't forced to reach for muscle tissue as the alternate supply of energy.

Carbohydrates are truly a double edged sword.

Although eliminating carbs does lead to the using of fat and muscle as alternate energy supplies, eating carbs **protects muscle tissue**, thereby forcing the burning of fat rather than muscle.

*The balance is a **real** struggle:*

Too many carbs and your body won't burn fat. Too little carbs, and your body burns through your muscle tissue. But, don't worry. Soon you'll have everything you need to find the right balance for your body.

Quality of Carbs

There are two main types of carbohydrates, commonly referred to as "**simple carbs**" and "**complex carbs**." What defines the quality of a carbohydrate is the speed at which it is absorbed – the rate at which your body breaks them down for use as energy.

Simple Carbohydrates

When carbohydrates are absorbed quickly (when simple carbohydrates are consumed), there is a quick bodily reaction of elevated blood sugar, which causes the brain to release the hormone **insulin** to get the body's blood sugar levels back under control.

The resulting danger is that when insulin is set in motion to regulate blood sugar, the hormone glucagon (the hormone that asks the body to use fat as an energy supply) is halted until the insulin has finished its work. Your body regulates the blood sugar while fat burning is suppressed.

Another common negative attribute of "simple" or *fast-absorbing carbohydrates* is that giving your body that high elevation in blood sugar results in an equally low swing in the opposite direction. Basically, after insulin kicks in and lowers your blood sugar, then your body craves food to push it back up.

You feel hungry quickly.
The long-term result is a complete loss of control in the way we handle our food. We over-eat, and we crave the same unhealthy carbohydrates that gave us the rush in the first place.

Regulating your carbohydrate intake is largely about regulating blood sugar levels to keep them at a balanced level.

Some examples of simple carbohydrates are: Baked goods, cookies, sugar, cereal, corn syrup, fruit juice concentrate, and dairy products.

Complex Carbohydrates

Complex carbohydrates are those that cause smaller increases in blood sugar because they take more time for the body to break down and use (they have longer chains of sugar molecules). They allow glucose to release into the blood stream slowly and consistently.

You want to fill as much of your carbohydrate intake with complex carbohydrates as possible.

Some great complex carbs are brown rice, whole wheat bread, yams, broccoli, carrots, pasta, quinoa, grains, beans, and fiber rich fruits.

Fiber is an interesting complex carbohydrate worth noting because it slows down the rate at which your body absorbs of other types of carbohydrates. Fiber is also indigestible, meaning that your body completely gets rid of it after its been made proper use of.

The Glycemic Index

The glycemic index is a scale that rates foods that can be categorized as carbohydrates based on the effect in the rise of blood sugar that the food has. Generally speaking, the higher the glycemic index rating (which is anywhere from 1 – 100), the more "simple" the carbohydrate is.

To get the most out of the carbohydrates you consume, try checking where the carbs you eat fall on this scale. The goal is to eat foods that fall ideally from 1-40 on the scale the majority of the time, and 40-75 sparingly.

GLYCEMIC INDEX CHART
LOW GLYCEMIC (55 OR BELOW)   HIGH GLYCEMIC (70 OR HIGHER)

SNACKS	G.I.	STARCH	G.I.	VEGETABLES	G.I.	FRUITS	G.I.	DAIRY	G.I.
PIZZA	33	BAGEL, PLAIN	33	BROCCOLI	10	CHERRIES	22	YOGURT, PLAIN	14
CHOCOLATE BAR	49	WHITE RICE	38	PEPPER	10	APPLE	38	YOGURT, LOW FAT	14
POUND CAKE	54	WHITE SPAGHETTI	58	LETTUCE	10	ORANGE	43	WHOLE MILK	30
POPCORN	55	SWEET POTATO	44	MUSHROOMS	10	GRAPES	46	SOY MILK	31
ENERGY BAR	58	WHITE BREAD	49	ONIONS	10	KIWI	52	SKIM MILK	32
SODA	72	BROWN RICE	55	GREEN PEAS	48	BANANA	56	CHOCOLATE MILK	35
DOUGHNUT	76	PANCAKES	67	CARROTS	49	PINEAPPLE	66	YOGURT, FRUIT	36
JELLY BEANS	80	WHEAT BREAD	80	BEETS	64	WATERMELON	72	CUSTARD	43
PRETZELS	83	BAKED POTATO	85	ONIONS	75	DATES	103	ICE CREAM	60

In Summary

1. Eliminating carbs is not the answer to a great body, although it can help you achieve rapid weight loss.

2. The body prefers carbohydrates as its main source of energy. Carbohydrates are converted into glucose and used as energy for bodily functions and processes.

3. You can cause your body to use fat and protein as a source of energy by regulating your carbohydrate intake.

4. Carbohydrates protect your muscle tissue from being used as energy, so it is important to find the right portion of carbohydrates to eat.

5. Simple carbohydrates cause rapid increases in blood sugar, which stops your body from burning fat and leaves you feeling hungry.

6. Fill your carbohydrate intake with complex carbohydrates like yams, brown rice, whole wheat bread, grains, vegetables, quinoa, fiber-rich fruits, and beans.

7. The glycemic index rates the complexity of carbohydrates based on the way they affect blood sugar levels after consumption.

8. The lower on the glycemic index scale a carbohydrate falls, the better it is for fat loss.

Proteins & Fats

Proteins

You have over 10,000 different proteins in your body. It is absolutely essential to every cell in the body. Protein is made up of amino acids, which, in relation to weight loss, are important in that they **grow and repair our muscle tissue.**

It is essential to consume enough protein because it helps keep you full, stimulates muscle growth, facilitates muscle retention, and it has a significant affect on our basal metabolic rate – the automatic functioning of our metabolism.

The more protein you eat, the faster your metabolism works. The faster your metabolism works, the more calories you naturally burn.

The mechanics of the way protein affects the metabolism are relatively simple.

Protein enlarges muscles if paired with exercise by adding additional proteins to muscle fibers. That process requires amino acids. When you eat more amino acids, which are what protein is made up of, it has a direct affect on muscle mass.

Increasing your muscle mass has an affect on the amount of calories you naturally burn because muscle tissue requires more energy than fat.

The more muscle you have and the less fat present in your body, the faster your metabolism operates.

It's been said a few times already fat loss is achieved by forcing the body to burn fat as a result of a caloric deficit. We've also said that the body turns not only to fat, but to muscle when it has energy requirements it needs to fulfill.

Although eating a certain amount of carbohydrates can curb the use of muscle tissue as an energy source, it is really important to continue to fill the body with protein to maintain the muscle in your body. Eating protein ensures that you continue to burn fat while keeping your muscle.

Another benefit of heavier protein consumption is that your body takes longer to digest, which requires the use of more energy in the process, and protein keeps you full for long periods of time.

When you eat a lot of protein with few carbohydrates, the metabolism changes and is placed into a state of **Ketosis**, which is another word to describe the process of burning fat rather than carbohydrates as an energy source.

Some great sources of protein include cottage cheese, eggs, steak, lean chicken, turkey, fish, beans, lentils, quinoa, protein and nuts.

Fats

Your body requires you to eat fat in order to burn fat. It is indispensable to eat some forms of healthy fats. **Essential fats** keep your skin and hair healthy, and are integral to hormone production.

"Good fats" are titled "essential" because the body can't produce them on its own, or work properly without them. They're also important for brain development, and controlling inflammation in the body.

"Bad fats" or "saturated/trans fats" have no true nutritional value and in fact harm the basic processes they're meant to help facilitate.

Healthy fat consumption can come from vegetable oils, all sorts of nuts, avocados, eggs, chia seeds, fatty fish, coconuts (in addition to coconut oil), peanut butter, seeds, greek yogurt, and even dark chocolate.

In Summary:

1. The more protein you fill your muscles through protein consumption, the faster your metabolism works.
2. Protein helps ensure you burn fat while retaining muscle.
3. Protein keeps you full for longer periods of time, and keeps the digestive process active.
4. You need to eat fat to burn fat, but it's important to refrain from eating saturated fat or trans-fat.
5. Nuts are the easiest and best way to consume the fat you need in your diet.

Taking Action On Your Nutrition Goals

At this point, most people will take a mental note on these dietary / food points to apply going forward. But in order to **guarantee our results,** we must **guarantee we'll take action on this every day**.

As powerful as mindsets are, they are also very malleable and easily influenced by outside stimuli (like having a very common "off day"). Meanwhile, systems (which provide accountability and tracking) are black and white - yes or no - 1 or 0.

We highly recommend putting together a structure you think can work in helping you stay consistent with your eating goals. Nothing is more demoralizing than aiming to feel better about yourself, working out hard for it, and seeing poor results (that you later justify).

After getting some clarity on which eating plan you want to follow (i.e. counting calories/macros or choosing a specific diet), there are a few ways to put it into effect.

As a free option

You can use a dietary tracking app, google sheet, or notepad to track calories/macros/meals. Alternatively you can use an extra whiteboard or calendar to track whether you hit your goals or not every day. If you think you can genuinely stay consistent with this for months / the long term, this is a great option.

As a paid option

Co-authors of this journal, Habit Nest, wrote the *The Nutrition Sidekick Journal* to help you nail down your diet - by providing a clear, unbreakable system to track your results and help you learn how to improve (without judgement!) at the same time.

If a pure tracking sheet is a bit too dull, redundant, and isn't stimulating enough for you, this may be the right choice.

Some things covered inside:

1. How to manipulate your body to burn fat while maintaining muscle
2. Tracking for your calories, water intake, and planned meals vs. actual eaten meals
3. New golden nuggets of information, pro-tips, daily challenges, and more each day

You can check it out at **SidekickJournal.com/Nutrition** and use discount code **BadassBooty15** for 15% off if you decide to order one.

Effectively Tracking Your Progress

Tracking your progress is extremely important. That being said, the accuracy of your tracking is **even more important**. With flawed data that isn't actionable, your tracking is just an arbitrary, confusing, and often misleading number.

This section assumes you have two body-composition goals, which tend to be the most popular amongst people (and can be the healthiest)

1. You want to increase your muscle mass
2. You want to reach & maintain your body fat percentage at 5-15% (males) or 10-20% (females)

If the above is true, as a general guideline your goal should first be to get as lean as you'd like, then switch to a *very slight* caloric surplus to build muscle in the long-term.

The problem with the scale

With weight training and fat loss, the scale's results (without deeper insight on it) can be your biggest enemy. This is because our shifts in bodyweight are affected by SO many factors, it's impossible to identify what has changed week by week with only a weight amount.

This is where **body fat tracking** comes in, right alongside **body weight tracking**. By combining the tracking of BOTH your body fat AND the scale, you're able to see exactly HOW your weight changed from week to week - whether you gained muscle, gained body fat, lost muscle, or lost body fat.

Measuring your body fat percentage accurately

There are many ways to do this, but the most cost-effective and practical way is to use a self-testing skinfold caliper. The one we recommend is the Accu-Measure as it costs roughly $6.50 on Amazon and has an existing scientific study backing up its effectiveness (it's within 1.1% accuracy of using an underwater body fat measurement, which is one of the highest levels of accuracy we have for measuring body fat).

Disclaimer: we have no affiliation with the Accu-Measure and aren't getting paid in any way for this recommendation. It's simply a great tool.

With the upsides being ease of use and cost, the biggest downsides of this method are the **potential inaccuracy** if you don't know how to measure yourself properly each week. Although it's **very possible to be incredibly accurate** with this method... it takes a good deal of practice. Thankfully the product comes with step-by-step guide that lays out how to use it as accurately as possible.

As long as you are measuring yourself in the same location weekly, even if your placement isn't perfect, you'll be able to have comparable results you trust week after week. Make your main goal in measuring be *consistency in measuring*.

How do I get the right data?

We recommend measuring yourself weekly for both body weight (with a scale) and body fat (with the Accu-Measure).

We want to eliminate as many factors that can cause data inconsistencies as possible. When taking your measurements, do it:

- At the same time of day (ideally mornings)
- With the same food/water intake that day (ideally none, do it right as you wake up)
- With the same amount of clothes on, and
- Without holding any objects that could throw your readings off (i.e. your phone)

You can write this data down as you progress through the journal (turn the page!) or record it on a note on your phone. If you choose the latter, make sure you don't hold your phone as you're measuring yourself.

Common misunderstandings with the Accu-Measure

After using the Accu-Measure ourselves, a few things were a bit unclear from the instruction sheet they provided. We spoke with a rep on the phone who helped clarify these points for us:

1. Where is the iliac crest?
To find your iliac crest, it should be near your waist line (like where you wear a belt) and you feel a big bone protruding out, towards the side of your body.

2. How can you measure consistently and accurately?
If you place the caliper directly on your skin, the ends will measure 2.5 inches exactly. You can use this to consistently grab the same distance each measurement.

Once you have grabbed your skin fold with your thumb and index finger, position the caliper halfway between the back of your skinfold (point closest to your body) and the front of the skinfold (point furthest from your body), 1cm away from your fingers.

Getting even more clarity, reducing measuring inaccuracy

The most important thing with using the Accu-Measure is **measuring yourself the same way week-to-week**. Even if you're measuring yourself improperly, or the Accu-Measure is inaccurate itself, your **week-to-week changes should remain consistent** as the method of measuring is consistent.

If you want to take this to the next level, or see how close to accurate your Accu-Measure is, you can get a detailed body scan (i.e. a $45 DEXA scan or water displacement scan) and see how it compares to the Accu-Measure. If a discrepancy exists, you'll at least know by how much and be able to mentally keep that in mind.

Write down the following each week

1. Measure your **total body weight** using a scale

2. Measure your **body fat %** using an Accu-Measure

3. Take your total body weight (#1) in pounds and multiply it by your body fat % (#2). This will give you your **body fat weight**.

4. Take your **total body weight** (#1) and subtract your **body fat weight** (#3) to get your **lean body mass**.

Your lean body mass consists of every part of your body that's not considered fat (muscles, tissues, bones, organs, water weight, etc.) Since a significant changing factor in weight of your lean body mass is your muscle mass, we can use lean body mass as a near-accurate measure of fluctuations in muscle gain / loss.

The biggest inconsistency with your lean body mass will be the fluctuations in your water weight. Be mindful of this and how certain factors (i.e. being dehydrated, drinking lots of water, intaking too much sodium the day before) can affect this. If something seems wrong, give it at least 2 weeks before jumping to conclusions of whether your plan is or is not working.

What should I do with this measurement data?

The next two pages provide a space to record this data weekly over a 12 week period, followed by actions steps for how to adjust weekly for each scenario.

Having this data recorded next to each other will allow you to spot trends in your weekly fluctuations and make the correct adjustments of action steps based on this.

Adjusting Based On Your Progress

As recommended in Tom Venuto's *Burn The Fat, Feed The Muscle*, you should make the following tweaks based on your weekly fluctuations of **body fat weight (B.F. Weight)** and **lean body mass (L.B.M.)** to achieve body fat loss & muscle gain:

1. **If:** | B.F. Weight (↑) | L.B.M. (↑) |

Then: Decrease your caloric intake (recommended: 100-200) and increase your cardio.

2. **If:** | B.F. Weight (↓) | L.B.M. (↑) |

Then: This is the holy grail and we are all jealous of you. Keep doing what you're doing. This is decently rare to occur, so treat it as a huge gift if you're lucky to experiencing it!

3. **If:** | B.F. Weight (↑) | L.B.M. (↓) |

Then: This is unlikely and usually due to a measurement inaccuracy. Alternatively, this may be due to factors outside of your training and nutrition, such as being under a lot of stress and not getting adequate rest. Recheck your results, and if they're accurate, take care of yourself and see if you notice a significant difference the following week.

4. **If:** | B.F. Weight (↓) | L.B.M. (↓) |

Then: Eat more calories (recommended: 100-200) and increase protein intake if you're under 1g * your total body weight.
Increasing your weight training intensity will help as well here.

5. **If:** | B.F. Weight (↑) | L.B.M. (—) | (This icon means "stayed the same")

Then: Eat less calories (recommended: 100-200) and slightly increase your cardio.
Note: This action step also applies if both your L.B.M. and your body fat weight stay the same (no change as the week before).

6. **If:** | B.F. Weight (↓) | L.B.M. (—) |

Then: This is fantastic! You're right on track, keep doing what you're doing.

Weekly Progress Tracker

WEEK 1
DATE: _____

WEIGHT: _____ BODY FAT %: _____

FAT WEIGHT: _____ LEAN BODY MASS: _____

ADJUSTMENTS TO MAKE
(CIRCLE)   (FILL IN AMOUNT)

CALORIES	↑	↓	—	_____
CARDIO	↑	↓	—	_____
TRAINING INTENSITY	↑	↓	—	

WEEK 2
DATE: _____

WEIGHT: _____ BODY FAT %: _____

FAT WEIGHT: _____ LEAN BODY MASS: _____

ADJUSTMENTS TO MAKE
(CIRCLE)   (FILL IN AMOUNT)

CALORIES	↑	↓	—	_____
CARDIO	↑	↓	—	_____
TRAINING INTENSITY	↑	↓	—	

WEEK 3
DATE: _____

WEIGHT: _____ BODY FAT %: _____

FAT WEIGHT: _____ LEAN BODY MASS: _____

ADJUSTMENTS TO MAKE
(CIRCLE)   (FILL IN AMOUNT)

CALORIES	↑	↓	—	_____
CARDIO	↑	↓	—	_____
TRAINING INTENSITY	↑	↓	—	

WEEK 4
DATE: _____

WEIGHT: _____ BODY FAT %: _____

FAT WEIGHT: _____ LEAN BODY MASS: _____

ADJUSTMENTS TO MAKE
(CIRCLE)   (FILL IN AMOUNT)

CALORIES	↑	↓	—	_____
CARDIO	↑	↓	—	_____
TRAINING INTENSITY	↑	↓	—	

WEEK 5
DATE: _____

WEIGHT: _____ BODY FAT %: _____

FAT WEIGHT: _____ LEAN BODY MASS: _____

ADJUSTMENTS TO MAKE
(CIRCLE)   (FILL IN AMOUNT)

CALORIES	↑	↓	—	_____
CARDIO	↑	↓	—	_____
TRAINING INTENSITY	↑	↓	—	

WEEK 6
DATE: _____

WEIGHT: _____ BODY FAT %: _____

FAT WEIGHT: _____ LEAN BODY MASS: _____

ADJUSTMENTS TO MAKE
(CIRCLE)   (FILL IN AMOUNT)

CALORIES	↑	↓	—	_____
CARDIO	↑	↓	—	_____
TRAINING INTENSITY	↑	↓	—	

WEEK 7

DATE: _____

WEIGHT: _____ BODY FAT %: _____

FAT WEIGHT: _____ LEAN BODY MASS: _____

ADJUSTMENTS TO MAKE

(CIRCLE)　　　　(FILL IN AMOUNT)

CALORIES　　↑　↓　—　_____

CARDIO　　↑　↓　—　_____

TRAINING INTENSITY　　↑　↓　—

WEEK 8

DATE: _____

WEIGHT: _____ BODY FAT %: _____

FAT WEIGHT: _____ LEAN BODY MASS: _____

ADJUSTMENTS TO MAKE

(CIRCLE)　　　　(FILL IN AMOUNT)

CALORIES　　↑　↓　—　_____

CARDIO　　↑　↓　—　_____

TRAINING INTENSITY　　↑　↓　—

WEEK 9

DATE: _____

WEIGHT: _____ BODY FAT %: _____

FAT WEIGHT: _____ LEAN BODY MASS: _____

ADJUSTMENTS TO MAKE

(CIRCLE)　　　　(FILL IN AMOUNT)

CALORIES　　↑　↓　—　_____

CARDIO　　↑　↓　—　_____

TRAINING INTENSITY　　↑　↓　—

WEEK 10

DATE: _____

WEIGHT: _____ BODY FAT %: _____

FAT WEIGHT: _____ LEAN BODY MASS: _____

ADJUSTMENTS TO MAKE

(CIRCLE)　　　　(FILL IN AMOUNT)

CALORIES　　↑　↓　—　_____

CARDIO　　↑　↓　—　_____

TRAINING INTENSITY　　↑　↓　—

Goal-Setting Principles

Whether you're working towards fitness goals, or other personal goals to improve the quality of your life, the process of creating a lasting change is multi-faceted.

It boils down to:

1. Having a concrete goal you want to reach,
2. Creating a realistic action plan that'll take you towards your goal
3. Preparing mentally and emotionally for obstacles that will undoubtedly arise,
4. Utilizing a proper system of accountability,
5. Tracking your progress so you see the results and benefits you're gaining, and
6. Taking action daily.

In terms of creating the action plan, using a system of accountability, tracking your progress, and discussing many of the obstacles that will arise, we have you covered from A-Z.

But, even though the entire blueprint is laid out, nothing changes without your daily action and commitment to your goal!

Your brain has to change before your body can.

Why We Know This Program Works

Fitness and performance expert Jennifer Cohen, co-author of this book and and bestselling author of '*Strong Is The New Skinny*' & '*No Gym Required*' has trained hundreds of clients using the training method you're given here.

Even more importantly, she is an entrepreneur involved in several businesses, and a mother of two.

Jen continues to find the time every day to implement this routine to keep herself in great shape.

The program has been intricately designed to combat the results of our bodies storing fat in our stomachs, hips, thighs, and butts, and re-shaping these problem areas to achieve a toned, fit look.

Perfectionists, Tread Lightly.

Of course, ideally we want to workout consistently and quickly see the results we're after as soon as we begin any exercise regimen.

But sometimes there's a problem with shooting for perfection from the very start.

So often you see people getting caught up in finding 'the best workout routine,' or 'the best diet for weight loss' that they never end up acting on their goal.

But we're going to let you in on a little secret.

There's one simple concept that shatters all the best research, tips and strategies you can look for (that you'll be getting here anyways).

The best way to shape your booty and trim your waist to get those amazing results is…. to start and do something.

You start taking SOME action towards your goal on a daily basis.

Don't let the desire to reach perfection - your goal body - stop you from making sure you have a great workout TODAY.

The best way to get the body you want is by trying one method for achieving it; following one specific strategy that has been laid out, and doing it for a period of time consistently.

Nobody else can do your workouts for you. All they can do is give you information.

It's up to YOU to try the program, learn what you can, see how effective it is, and only then make an educated choice about how to move forward.

You'll be getting all the information and motivation you need from us on a daily basis in the workouts you're getting.

If you make use of every workout to just take a small step towards your goal, you WILL see the results you're after. Pinky promise.

Because every little action you take in the direction of your goals propels a snowball effect that greatly impacts other areas of your life.

If you push yourself to do this program for even 1 week, you're gifting yourself a positive chain of effects that will improve your daily energy, mental clarity, and increase your self-confidence.

In turn, if you don't prioritize your workouts, each of these benefits gets sacrificed.

Break through every obstacle you may face to absolutely get your workout done TODAY.

And then repeat.

Because success is all about taking small, consistent actions over time.

Developing Strength From The Inside Out

Your head can be your friend or foe when it comes to getting stronger, fitter, and sexier.

That's because your mind is your most powerful muscle, so you can either flex it to boost your motivation and perseverance (which is great) or clench it to resist your efforts (which is bad).

Our advice is to pick option number one.

Here is what you stand to gain: A stronger, more consistent sense of motivation, a can-do spirit, a clearer vision of your goals and the mental clarity and fortitude to reach them.

So ask yourself, is your mind your ally or enemy when it comes to getting fit?

When you think about your body - its state, its shape, and its capabilities - do your thoughts sound more like the hip, cool captain of your own cheerleading squad or more like an abusive prison guard?

If it's the latter, it's time to evict that critical, sadistic voice and replace it with a more positive one.

The key is to change the way you think and talk about your body; if you don't have anything nice to say, shut up already!

Seriously, it's time to reclaim your mind and put it to good use for your body's sake.

If you've already got an upbeat mind, you can kick up your mental strength and positivity a notch or two and take it to the next level.

The truth is that you can talk yourself into or out of anything, so why not steer yourself in a positive direction?

Cranking up the strength in your head while you're ramping up your physical strength will produce a win-win outcome:

> *The mental vigor you'll be developing will fuel your physical fitness and vice versa, creating an awesome mind-body synergy that will help you grow and thrive and become the best version of yourself yet.*

When you condition your body to overcome hurdles or bounce back from setbacks, you will encourage your mind to do the same. It's a two-way street.

You Are Perfect As You Are

In going through this process, it's really important to keep in mind that you are already perfect, and that increasing your confidence and becoming a healthier you has nothing to do with your innate quality as a human being.

Looking or not looking a certain way does not make you inferior or superior to anyone else. Exercise and healthy eating are an essential part of living a well-rounded, healthy life.

It is objectively related to your health, well-being and weight loss.

Your end goal here isn't to be a certain weight or look a certain way, **it's to increase the quality of your emotional relationship with yourself.** You want to increase your energy levels, confidence, acceptance and ultimately love for yourself.

Never forget that changing your body through exercise and diet is simply a vehicle for that. If you can get there regardless of food, you've won the true battle.

What Are You Waiting For?

Everybody knows what his or her personal best is, and if you are not there or anywhere near it in terms of looking and feeling the way you want to, you have to ask yourself, "what am I waiting for?"

You (hopefully) just learned a lot about booty-building, torching fat through exercise and diet, and how we're going to help you attain your fitness goals.

But even though the blueprint for the plan is completely laid out and you have all the tools you need for hitting your goal, you have to remember that this whole process starts *and* ends with you.

Your job is to commit to the plan - mentally, physically, and emotionally until you realize that you can and will reach your goal with the right attitude.

With an attitude that is dead set on reaching the goal you set out to accomplish, literally nothing can stop you.

General Safety Tips

For All Days:

1. If you begin feeling any pain, do NOT continue with an exercise. Feel free to switch to any exercise that does not cause you pain.

2. You always want the muscle you're working on to take the load, not your back or other parts of the body - all it takes is ONE bad set, ONE bad rep to set you back weeks or even months.

3. Don't extent to the absolute limit of your flexibility unless you're extremely comfortable with the exercise.

4. Be aware of your surroundings. Make sure there's nothing you could knock over or can injure you during your workouts, especially ones with movement.

For Weight Training Days:

1. Never invent new uses for a machine!

2. When picking up weights, use proper form. Bend with your knees and use leg strength to pick up the weight. Avoids injury from straining back and hips.

3. If you're unsure of whether you can complete a rep for a workout where you can't just drop the weights, USE a ***spotter*** - someone to help you finish the movement if you get stuck.

4. Don't just drop weights, they fall hard and bounce around. You can hurt others or yourself when you drop the weights from your hands to the floor. Use a controlled movement to place weights on the ground or in their proper place.

5. Fingers and toes are weirdly susceptible to getting hurt when picking up or putting weights down - watch out for it. Ari once bruised his finger because he put the weight on the rack too quickly and the dumbbell went over the rack with his finger caught in between it and the rack.

6. If you've made the very normal mistake of using a weight that's too heavy for you and you realize you need help because you're in a situation in which you're not sure what to do - ASK for help from somebody nearby!!

7. Always be aware of your surroundings - make sure what you're doing doesn't jeopardize anybody else's safety.

Commit.

No matter what happens tomorrow...

*whether I am exhausted
or have the **worst** day of my life...*

*...whether I win the lottery
or have the **best** day of my life...*

*I **will** do my workout.*

*My word is like **gold**.*

*I will do whatever it takes
to make this happen.*

I will workout at least this many times this week (circle one):

1   2   3   4   5   6   7

_____   _____
Signature   Date

The Extreme Importance of Form

Before beginning any exercise, you have to be absolutely sure that you understand how to complete the exercise properly without getting injured.

We provide explanations of each exercise in the back of this journal, but if you're ever unclear, it only takes 30 seconds to look any exercise up online.

Our bodies are masters of compensation.

Where the body can 'cheat' by using more muscles than necessary to complete a movement, it will.

There must be a constant vigilance to retain proper form. And let's be very clear: Form is **vitally** important.

Without proper form:

1. There is always a *risk of injury.*
2. You're most likely *missing the target muscle* because you're *overcompensating with body parts that don't need to be used.*

There is never a good reason not to use proper form on any given exercise.

Workout 1: 4-3-2-1

HabitNest.link/booty01
EXERCISE GUIDE

DATE _____

GLUTE ACTIVATION WARMUP
 30s EACH

a. Clam Opener

(30s Each Side)

b. Glute Bridge w/ Band Flutter

c. Fire Hydrant

(30s Each Leg)

d. Lateral Leg Raise

- 30s Each Leg (w/ Foot Flexed)
- 30s Each Leg (w/ Toes Pointing Down)

——————— 30 SECOND BREAK ———————

CIRCUIT 1
 60s EACH

1a. Curtsy Lunge

REPS: _____
(Left Leg)

→

1b. Curtsy Lunge

REPS: _____
(Right Leg)

→

1c. Boxing Jab

REPS: _____

→

1d. Side to Side Squat

REPS: _____

——————— 30 SECOND BREAK ———————

CIRCUIT 2
50s EACH

2a. 180° Jump Twist to Floor Tap

SET 1 REPS: _____

SET 2 REPS: _____

→

2b. Squat w/ Overhead Press

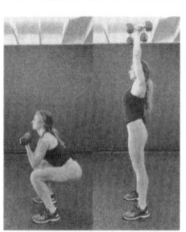

SET 1 REPS: _____

SET 2 REPS: _____

→

2c. Plie Jump Squat

SET 1 REPS: _____

SET 2 REPS: _____

─── 30 SECOND BREAK ───

 ## CIRCUIT 3

3a. Lateral Lunge to Reverse Lunge   ### 3b. Roundhouse Kick to Squat

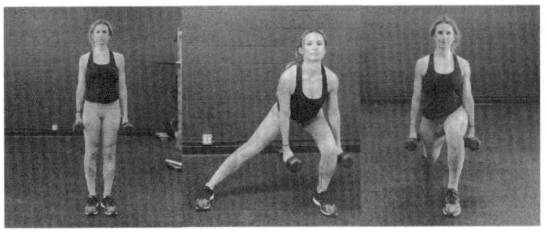

(Left Leg)   SET 1 REPS: _____   →   (Left Leg)   SET 1 REPS: _____
(Right Leg)   SET 2 REPS: _____   →   (Right Leg)   SET 2 REPS: _____
(Alternate Legs)   SET 3 REPS: _____   →   (Alternate Legs)   SET 3 REPS: _____

─── 30 SECOND BREAK ───

4a. Leap Forward into Squat, Burpee, Shuffle Back   ## CIRCUIT 4   (Reminder: If you feel pain with any exercise, STOP! Do NOT push through. Try a different exercise instead)

SET 1 REPS: _____ → 15s REST
SET 2 REPS: _____ → 15s REST
SET 3 REPS: _____ → 15s REST
SET 4 REPS: _____ → 15s REST

─── 30 SECOND BREAK ───

 ## COOL DOWN

a. Hamstring Stretch   **b. Glute Stretch**   **c. Pigeon Stretch**   **d. Runner's Stretch**

Workout 2: 4-3-2-1

HabitNest.link/booty02

DATE _____

GLUTE ACTIVATION WARMUP

a. Clam Opener

(30s Each Side)

b. Lateral Leg Raise

- 30s Each Leg (w/ Foot Flexed)
- 30s Each Leg (w/ Toes Pointing Down)

c. Glute Bridge w/ Leg Extension

(30s Each Leg)

d. Tabletop w/ Diagonal Kick

(30s Each Leg)

——— 30 SECOND BREAK ———

CIRCUIT 1

1a. Burpee

REPS: _____ →

1b. Reverse Dumbbell Fly

REPS: _____ →

1c. Mountain Climber

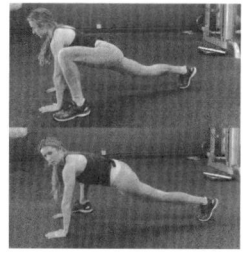

REPS: _____
(Alternate Sides) →

1d. Starfish Crunch

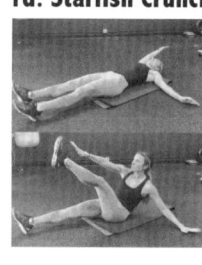

REPS: _____
(Alternate Sides)

——— 30 SECOND BREAK ———

CIRCUIT 2

2a. Jump Twist

SET 1 REPS: _____ →

SET 2 REPS: _____ →

2b. Plank to Row

SET 1 REPS: _____
(Alternate Sides) →

SET 2 REPS: _____
(Alternate Sides) →

2c. Vertical Sit-Up w/ Elbow to Knee Touch

SET 1 REPS: _____
(Alternate Sides)

SET 2 REPS: _____
(Alternate Sides)

———————————— 30 SECOND BREAK ————————————

 ## CIRCUIT 3

3a. Side Plank w/ Elbow Twist
3b. Fast Feet

(Left Side)   SET 1 REPS: _____ → SET 1 REPS: _____

(Right Side)   SET 2 REPS: _____ → SET 2 REPS: _____

(Alternate Sides)   SET 3 REPS: _____ → SET 3 REPS: _____

———————————— 30 SECOND BREAK ————————————

 ## CIRCUIT 4

4a. Squat to Overhead Press

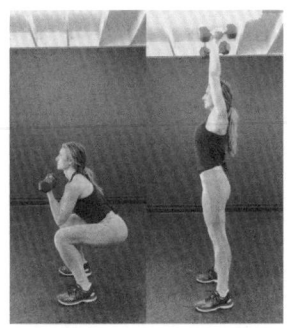

SET 1 REPS: _____ → 15s REST

SET 2 REPS: _____ → 15s REST

SET 3 REPS: _____ → 15s REST

SET 4 REPS: _____ → 15s REST

———————————— 30 SECOND BREAK ————————————

 ## COOL DOWN

a. Runner's Stretch   b. Butterfly Stretch   c. Lat Stretch   d. Crossbody Hangover

A quick note from our team:

Happy with your journal so far?

We worked very hard to build this - it would mean the absolute WORLD if you could share an honest review of your experience on Amazon with it.
HabitNest.link/bootyreview

Having any issues or problems?

This is one of our early runs of this journal - we know we have ways to improve it, so if you're having anything less than a 5-star experience PLEASE email us at mikey+booty@habitnest.com so we can learn how to improve / see what we can do for you.

Regardless, we won't rest until you have an incredible experience here... promise :)

With love,
Jennifer, Ari, Amir, & Mikey

Workout 3: Weight Training

HabitNest.link/booty03

EXERCISE GUIDE

DATE _____

1. Deadlift

SET 1   REPS: _____   (GOAL: 15-20)   WEIGHT: _____
SET 2   REPS: _____   (GOAL: 12-15)   WEIGHT: _____
SET 3   REPS: _____   (GOAL: 10-12)   WEIGHT: _____
SET 4   REPS: _____   (GOAL: 8-10)   WEIGHT: _____
(Optional)

2. Hip Thrust

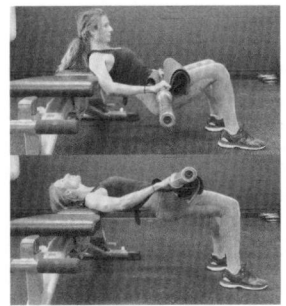

SET 1   REPS: _____   (GOAL: 15-20)   WEIGHT: _____
SET 2   REPS: _____   (GOAL: 12-15)   WEIGHT: _____
SET 3   REPS: _____   (GOAL: 10-12)   WEIGHT: _____
SET 4   REPS: _____   (GOAL: 8-10)   WEIGHT: _____
(Optional)

3. Squat

SET 1   REPS: _____   (GOAL: 15-20)   WEIGHT: _____
SET 2   REPS: _____   (GOAL: 12-15)   WEIGHT: _____
SET 3   REPS: _____   (GOAL: 10-12)   WEIGHT: _____
SET 4   REPS: _____   (GOAL: 8-10)   WEIGHT: _____
(Optional)

4. Alternating Step Up

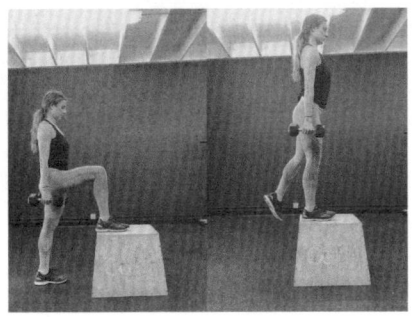

SET 1   REPS: _____   (GOAL: 15-20)   WEIGHT: _____
SET 2   REPS: _____   (GOAL: 12-15)   WEIGHT: _____
SET 3   REPS: _____   (GOAL: 10-12)   WEIGHT: _____
SET 4   REPS: _____   (GOAL: 8-10)   WEIGHT: _____
(Optional)

HabitNest.link/booty04

Workout 4: 4-3-2-1

DATE

 GLUTE ACTIVATION WARMUP

a. Double Walk Out **b. Box Draw** **c. Box Draw** **d. Running Man**

(2 Steps Right, 2 Steps Left) (Left Side) (Right Side) (30s Each Leg)

──── 30 SECOND BREAK ────

 CIRCUIT 1

1a. Burpee **1b. Bulgarian Lunge** **1c. Bulgarian Lunge** **1d. Mountain Climber**

REPS: _____ → REPS: _____ → REPS: _____ → REPS: _____
                (Right Leg)   (Left Leg)   (Alternate Sides)

──── 30 SECOND BREAK ────

 CIRCUIT 2

2a. Jump Lunge **2b. Single Leg Glute Bridge** **2c. Speed Skater**

SET 1 REPS: _____ → SET 1 REPS: _____ → SET 1 REPS: _____
(Alternate Legs)   (Left Leg)   (Alternate Sides)

SET 2 REPS: _____ → SET 2 REPS: _____ → SET 2 REPS: _____
(Alternate Legs)   (Right Leg)   (Alternate Sides)

──────── 30 SECOND BREAK ────────

CIRCUIT 3

3a. Russian Twist **3b. Side Shuffle w/ Floor Tap**

(Left Side)	SET 1 REPS: _____	→	SET 1 REPS: _____
(Right Side)	SET 2 REPS: _____	→	SET 2 REPS: _____
(Alternate Sides)	SET 3 REPS: _____	→	SET 3 REPS: _____

──────── 30 SECOND BREAK ────────

CIRCUIT 4

4a. Squat Jack

SET 1 REPS: _____ → 15s REST
SET 2 REPS: _____ → 15s REST
SET 3 REPS: _____ → 15s REST
SET 4 REPS: _____ → 15s REST

──────── 30 SECOND BREAK ────────

COOL DOWN

a. Hamstring Stretch   **b. Pigeon Stretch**   **c. Glute Stretch**   **d. Lat Stretch**

Psssstt... We like rewarding people (like you) who TAKE ACTION and actually use this journal.

Email us now at secret+booty@habitnest.com for a secret gift ;)

Workout 5: Weight Training

HabitNest.link/booty05
EXERCISE GUIDE

DATE _____

1. Shoulder Rope Pull

SET 1	REPS: _____	(GOAL: 15-20)	WEIGHT: _____
SET 2	REPS: _____	(GOAL: 12-15)	WEIGHT: _____
SET 3	REPS: _____	(GOAL: 10-12)	WEIGHT: _____
SET 4 (Optional)	REPS: _____	(GOAL: 8-10)	WEIGHT: _____

2. Lateral Raise

SET 1	REPS: _____	(GOAL: 15-20)	WEIGHT: _____
SET 2	REPS: _____	(GOAL: 12-15)	WEIGHT: _____
SET 3	REPS: _____	(GOAL: 10-12)	WEIGHT: _____
SET 4 (Optional)	REPS: _____	(GOAL: 8-10)	WEIGHT: _____

3. Straight Arm Rope Pull

SET 1	REPS: _____	(GOAL: 15-20)	WEIGHT: _____
SET 2	REPS: _____	(GOAL: 12-15)	WEIGHT: _____
SET 3	REPS: _____	(GOAL: 10-12)	WEIGHT: _____
SET 4 (Optional)	REPS: _____	(GOAL: 8-10)	WEIGHT: _____

4. Cable Row w/Squat

SET 1	REPS: _____	(GOAL: 15-20)	WEIGHT: _____
SET 2	REPS: _____	(GOAL: 12-15)	WEIGHT: _____
SET 3	REPS: _____	(GOAL: 10-12)	WEIGHT: _____
SET 4 (Optional)	REPS: _____	(GOAL: 8-10)	WEIGHT: _____

HabitNest.link/booty06

Workout 6: 4-3-2-1

 DATE

 GLUTE ACTIVATION WARMUP

a. Double Walk Out

(2 Steps Right, 2 Steps Left)

b. Box Draw

(Left Side)

c. Box Draw

(Right Side)

d. Running Man

(30s Each Leg)

─────── 30 SECOND BREAK ───────

 CIRCUIT 1

1a. Vertical Leap   **1b. Woodchopper**   **1b. Woodchopper**   **1d. The Heisman**

REPS: _____ → REPS: _____ → REPS: _____ → REPS: _____
                      (Right Side)   (Left Side)

─────── 30 SECOND BREAK ───────

 CIRCUIT 2

2a. Squat Thrust   **2b. Lateral Lunge to Curtsy Lunge**   **2c. Mountain Climber**

SET 1 REPS: _____ → SET 1 REPS: _____ → SET 1 REPS: _____
                           (Left Leg)   (Alternate Sides)

SET 2 REPS: _____ → SET 2 REPS: _____ → SET 2 REPS: _____
                           (Right Leg)   (Alternate Sides)

─── 30 SECOND BREAK ───

 CIRCUIT 3

3a. Lateral Lunge w/ Half 'X'

3b. 180° Jump Twist to Floor Tap

(Left Side)	SET 1 REPS: _____	→	SET 1 REPS: _____
(Right Side)	SET 2 REPS: _____	→	SET 2 REPS: _____
(Alternate Sides)	SET 3 REPS: _____	→	SET 3 REPS: _____

─── 30 SECOND BREAK ───

 CIRCUIT 4

4a. Leap Forward in Squat, Burpee, & Shuffle Back

SET 1 REPS: _____ → 15s REST
SET 2 REPS: _____ → 15s REST
SET 3 REPS: _____ → 15s REST
SET 4 REPS: _____ → 15s REST

─── 30 SECOND BREAK ───

 COOL DOWN

a. Hamstring Stretch   b. Crossbody Hangover   c. Runner's Stretch   d. Butterfly Stretch

EXERCISE GUIDE — HabitNest.link/booty07

Workout 7: 4-3-2-1

DATE _____

 GLUTE ACTIVATION WARMUP (30s EACH)

a. Clam Opener **b. Tabletop w/ Diagonal Kick** **c. Glute Bridge w/ Leg Extension** **d. Fire Hydrant**

(30s Each Side)   (30s Each Leg)   (30s Each Leg)   (30s Each Leg)

———————————— 30 SECOND BREAK ————————————

 CIRCUIT 1 (60s EACH)

1a. Jump Twist   **1b. Side Triangle Crunch**   **1c. Side Triangle Crunch**   **1d. Reverse Dumbbell Fly**

REPS: _____ → REPS: _____ (Right Side) → REPS: _____ (Left Side) → REPS: _____

———————————— 30 SECOND BREAK ————————————

 CIRCUIT 2 (50s EACH)

2a. Speed Skater   **2b. Plank to Row**   **2c. V-Up**

SET 1 REPS: _____ → SET 1 REPS: _____ (Alternate Arms) → SET 1 REPS: _____

SET 2 REPS: _____ → SET 2 REPS: _____ (Alternate Arms) → SET 2 REPS: _____

─── 30 SECOND BREAK ───

 ## CIRCUIT 3

3a. Spider-man Plank Crunch   ### 3b. Burpees

(Alternate Sides)   SET 1 REPS: _____   →   SET 1 REPS: _____

(Alternate Sides)   SET 2 REPS: _____   →   SET 2 REPS: _____

(Alternate Sides)   SET 3 REPS: _____   →   SET 3 REPS: _____

─── 30 SECOND BREAK ───

 ## CIRCUIT 4

4a. Ski Mogul

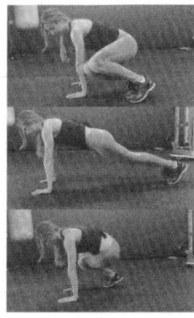

SET 1 REPS: _____   →   15s REST

SET 2 REPS: _____   →   15s REST

SET 3 REPS: _____   →   15s REST

SET 4 REPS: _____   →   15s REST

─── 30 SECOND BREAK ───

 ## COOL DOWN

a. Glute Stretch   ### b. Butterfly Stretch   ### c. Pigeon Stretch   ### d. Lat Stretch

Workout 8: Weight Training

HabitNest.link/booty08
EXERCISE GUIDE

DATE _____

1. Elevated Plie Squat

SET 1	REPS: _____	(GOAL: 15-20)	WEIGHT: _____
SET 2	REPS: _____	(GOAL: 12-15)	WEIGHT: _____
SET 3	REPS: _____	(GOAL: 10-12)	WEIGHT: _____
SET 4 (Optional)	REPS: _____	(GOAL: 8-10)	WEIGHT: _____

2. Woodchopper

Left | Right

SET 1	REPS: _____	_____ (GOAL: 15-20)	WEIGHT: _____
SET 2	REPS: _____	_____ (GOAL: 12-15)	WEIGHT: _____
SET 3	REPS: _____	_____ (GOAL: 10-12)	WEIGHT: _____
SET 4 (Optional)	REPS: _____	_____ (GOAL: 8-10)	WEIGHT: _____

3. Squat

SET 1	REPS: _____	(GOAL: 15-20)	WEIGHT: _____
SET 2	REPS: _____	(GOAL: 12-15)	WEIGHT: _____
SET 3	REPS: _____	(GOAL: 10-12)	WEIGHT: _____
SET 4 (Optional)	REPS: _____	(GOAL: 8-10)	WEIGHT: _____

4. Hip Thrust

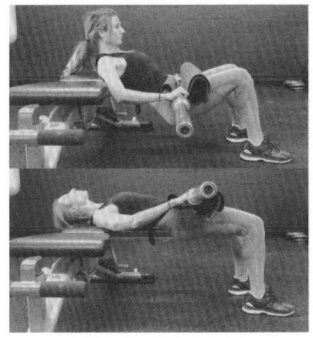

SET 1	REPS: _____	(GOAL: 15-20)	WEIGHT: _____
SET 2	REPS: _____	(GOAL: 12-15)	WEIGHT: _____
SET 3	REPS: _____	(GOAL: 10-12)	WEIGHT: _____
SET 4 (Optional)	REPS: _____	(GOAL: 8-10)	WEIGHT: _____

Workout 9: 4-3-2-1

HabitNest.link/booty09

DATE _____

 GLUTE ACTIVATION WARMUP (30s EACH)

a. Double Walk Out

(2 Steps Right, 2 Steps Left)

b. Box Draw

(Left Side)

c. Box Draw

(Right Side)

d. Running Man

(30s Each Leg)

——————— 30 SECOND BREAK ———————

 CIRCUIT 1 (60s EACH)

1a. High Knee

REPS: _____ →

1b. Bulgarian Lunge

REPS: _____
(Right Leg) →

1c. Bulgarian Lunge

REPS: _____
(Left Leg) →

1d. Side V-Up

REPS: _____
(30s Each Side)

——————— 30 SECOND BREAK ———————

 CIRCUIT 2 (50s EACH)

2a. Side Shuffle w/ Floor Tap

SET 1 REPS: _____ →
SET 2 REPS: _____ →

2b. Plank Step Up

SET 1 REPS: _____ →
SET 2 REPS: _____ →

2c. In and Out Jack

SET 1 REPS: _____
SET 2 REPS: _____

──── 30 SECOND BREAK ────

 CIRCUIT 3

3a. Side Plank w/ Torso Twist
3b. Lateral Lunge w/ Half 'X'

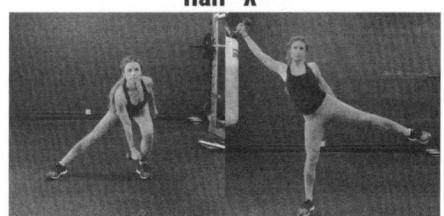

(Left Side)	SET 1 REPS: _____	→	(Left Side)	SET 1 REPS: _____
(Right Side)	SET 2 REPS: _____	→	(Right Side)	SET 2 REPS: _____
(Alternate Side)	SET 3 REPS: _____	→	(Alternate Side)	SET 3 REPS: _____

──── 30 SECOND BREAK ────

 CIRCUIT 4

4a. Pendulum Jack

SET 1 REPS: _____ → 15s REST
SET 2 REPS: _____ → 15s REST
SET 3 REPS: _____ → 15s REST
SET 4 REPS: _____ → 15s REST

──── 30 SECOND BREAK ────

 COOL DOWN

a. Hamstring Stretch **b. Runner's Stretch** **c. Butterfly Stretch** **d. Lat Stretch**

EXERCISE GUIDE — HabitNest.link/booty10

Workout 10: Weight Training

DATE: _____

1. Reverse Dumbbell Fly

SET 1	REPS: _____	(GOAL: 15-20)	WEIGHT: _____
SET 2	REPS: _____	(GOAL: 12-15)	WEIGHT: _____
SET 3	REPS: _____	(GOAL: 10-12)	WEIGHT: _____
SET 4 (Optional)	REPS: _____	(GOAL: 8-10)	WEIGHT: _____

2. Shoulder Rope Pull

SET 1	REPS: _____	(GOAL: 15-20)	WEIGHT: _____
SET 2	REPS: _____	(GOAL: 12-15)	WEIGHT: _____
SET 3	REPS: _____	(GOAL: 10-12)	WEIGHT: _____
SET 4 (Optional)	REPS: _____	(GOAL: 8-10)	WEIGHT: _____

3. Lateral Raise

SET 1	REPS: _____	(GOAL: 15-20)	WEIGHT: _____
SET 2	REPS: _____	(GOAL: 12-15)	WEIGHT: _____
SET 3	REPS: _____	(GOAL: 10-12)	WEIGHT: _____
SET 4 (Optional)	REPS: _____	(GOAL: 8-10)	WEIGHT: _____

4. Arnold Press

SET 1	REPS: _____	(GOAL: 15-20)	WEIGHT: _____
SET 2	REPS: _____	(GOAL: 12-15)	WEIGHT: _____
SET 3	REPS: _____	(GOAL: 10-12)	WEIGHT: _____
SET 4 (Optional)	REPS: _____	(GOAL: 8-10)	WEIGHT: _____

Check-In

Taking a few minutes to simply STOP and evaluate how you're doing mentally, physically, and emotionally every few weeks of a training program can be extremely helpful to your experience with the program.

Take a few minutes to answer the following questions with honesty!

What is my goal in completing this process - how do I want to look, feel, and what do I expect from doing this?

How am I ACTUALLY feeling physically?

_____
_____
_____
_____

How am I feeling about the quality and intensity of my workouts? Can I do more or am I pushing the limit consistently? Am I getting enough rest?

_____
_____
_____
_____

How do I feel about the way I look? Do I see how much I can change if I stick to this program?

_____
_____
_____
_____

What do I want to learn about this process that I can spend some time researching?

_____
_____
_____
_____

HabitNest.link/booty11
EXERCISE GUIDE

Workout 11: 4-3-2-1

DATE _____

GLUTE ACTIVATION WARMUP (30s EACH)

a. Clam Opener

(30s Each Side)

b. Glute Bridge w/ Band Flutter

c. Fire Hydrant

(30s Each Side)

d. Lateral Leg Raise

- 30s Each Leg (w/ Foot Flexed)
- 30s Each Leg (w/ Toes Pointing Down)

———— 30 SECOND BREAK ————

CIRCUIT 1 (60s EACH)

1a. Vertical Leap

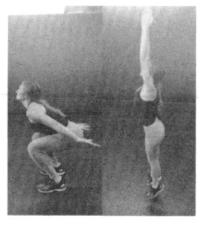

REPS: _____

→

1b. Lateral Lunge to Curtsy Lunge

REPS: _____
(Right Side)

→

1c. Lateral Lunge to Curtsy Lunge

REPS: _____
(Left Side)

→

1d. Squat Thrust

REPS: _____

———— 30 SECOND BREAK ————

CIRCUIT 2 (50s EACH)

2a. Russian Twist

SET 1 REPS: _____

SET 2 REPS: _____

→

2b. Plie Jump Squat

SET 1 REPS: _____

SET 2 REPS: _____

→

2c. Ski Mogul

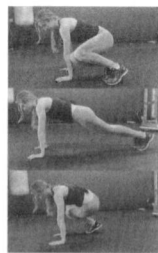

SET 1 REPS: _____

SET 2 REPS: _____

--- 30 SECOND BREAK ---

CIRCUIT 3

3a. Roundhouse Kick to Squat   3b. Leg Drop

(Left Leg)   SET 1 REPS: _____   →   SET 1 REPS: _____
(Right Leg)   SET 2 REPS: _____   →   SET 2 REPS: _____
(Alternate Legs)   SET 3 REPS: _____   →   SET 3 REPS: _____

--- 30 SECOND BREAK ---

CIRCUIT 4

4a. Burpee

SET 1 REPS: _____   →   15s REST
SET 2 REPS: _____   →   15s REST
SET 3 REPS: _____   →   15s REST
SET 4 REPS: _____   →   15s REST

--- 30 SECOND BREAK ---

COOL DOWN

a. Hamstring Stretch   **b. Pigeon Stretch**   **c. Lat Stretch**   **d. Butterfly Stretch**

HabitNest.link/booty12
EXERCISE GUIDE

Workout 12: 4-3-2-1

DATE _____

GLUTE ACTIVATION WARMUP
(30s EACH)

a. Clam Opener **b. Glute Bridge w/ Band Flutter** **c. Tabletop w/Donkey Kick** **d. Lateral Leg Raise**

(30s Each Side)

- 30s Each Leg (w/ Foot Flexed)
- 30s Each Leg (w/ Toes Pointing Down)

———————— 30 SECOND BREAK ————————

 ## CIRCUIT 1
(60s EACH)

1a. Mountain Climber **1b. Side V-Up** **1c. Side V-Up** **1d. High Knee**

REPS: _____ → REPS: _____ → REPS: _____ → REPS: _____
                    (Right Side)   (Left Side)

———————— 30 SECOND BREAK ————————

 ## CIRCUIT 2
(50s EACH)

2a. Starfish Crunch **2b. Plank Step Up** **2c. Woodchopper**

SET 1 REPS: _____ → SET 1 REPS: _____ → SET 1 REPS: _____
(Alternate Arms)   (Alternate Arms)   (Left Side)

SET 2 REPS: _____ → SET 2 REPS: _____ → SET 2 REPS: _____
(Alternate Arms)   (Alternate Arms)   (Right Side)

———————————— 30 SECOND BREAK ————————————

CIRCUIT 3

3a. Plie Squat w/ Shoulder Windmill

3b. The Heisman

SET 1 REPS: _____ → SET 1 REPS: _____

SET 2 REPS: _____ → SET 2 REPS: _____

SET 3 REPS: _____ → SET 3 REPS: _____

———————————— 30 SECOND BREAK ————————————

CIRCUIT 4

4a. 180° Jump Twist to Floor Tap

SET 1 REPS: _____ → (15s) REST

SET 2 REPS: _____ → (15s) REST

SET 3 REPS: _____ → (15s) REST

SET 4 REPS: _____ → (15s) REST

———————————— 30 SECOND BREAK ————————————

COOL DOWN

a. Pigeon Stretch   **b. Hamstring Stretch**   **c. Lat Stretch**   **d. Glute Stretch**

Workout 13: Weight Training

HabitNest.link/booty13
EXERCISE GUIDE

DATE _____

1. Single Leg Deadlift

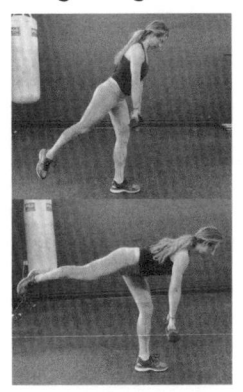

	Left	Right		
SET 1	REPS: _____	_____	(GOAL: 15-20)	WEIGHT: _____
SET 2	REPS: _____	_____	(GOAL: 12-15)	WEIGHT: _____
SET 3	REPS: _____	_____	(GOAL: 10-12)	WEIGHT: _____
SET 4 (Optional)	REPS: _____	_____	(GOAL: 8-10)	WEIGHT: _____

2. Single Leg Glute Bridge

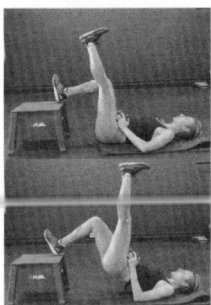

	Left	Right		
SET 1	REPS: _____	_____	(GOAL: 15-20)	WEIGHT: _____
SET 2	REPS: _____	_____	(GOAL: 12-15)	WEIGHT: _____
SET 3	REPS: _____	_____	(GOAL: 10-12)	WEIGHT: _____
SET 4 (Optional)	REPS: _____	_____	(GOAL: 8-10)	WEIGHT: _____

3. Squat

SET 1	REPS: _____	(GOAL: 15-20)	WEIGHT: _____
SET 2	REPS: _____	(GOAL: 12-15)	WEIGHT: _____
SET 3	REPS: _____	(GOAL: 10-12)	WEIGHT: _____
SET 4 (Optional)	REPS: _____	(GOAL: 8-10)	WEIGHT: _____

4. Hip Thrust

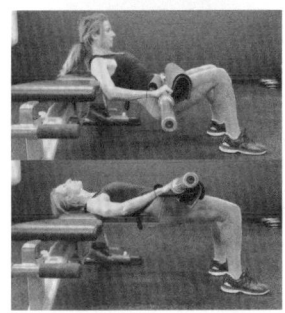

SET 1	REPS: _____	(GOAL: 15-20)	WEIGHT: _____
SET 2	REPS: _____	(GOAL: 12-15)	WEIGHT: _____
SET 3	REPS: _____	(GOAL: 10-12)	WEIGHT: _____
SET 4 (Optional)	REPS: _____	(GOAL: 8-10)	WEIGHT: _____

Workout 14: 4-3-2-1

HabitNest.link/booty14

DATE _____

GLUTE ACTIVATION WARMUP (30s EACH)

a. Double Walk Out

(2 Steps Right, 2 Steps Left)

b. Box Draw

(Left Side)

c. Box Draw

(Right Side)

d. Tabletop w/Donkey Kick

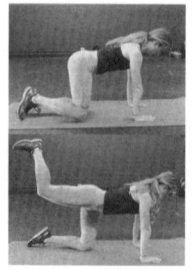

(30s Each Leg)

———— 30 SECOND BREAK ————

CIRCUIT 1 (60s EACH)

1a. Plie Jump Squat

REPS: _____ →

1b. Lateral Lunge w/ Half 'X'

REPS: _____
(Right Side) →

1c. Lateral Lunge w/ Half 'X'

REPS: _____
(Left Side) →

1d. Spider-man Plank Crunch

REPS: _____
(Alternate Sides)

———— 30 SECOND BREAK ————

CIRCUIT 2 (50s EACH)

2a. Standing Side Crunch

SET 1 REPS: _____
(Left Side)

SET 2 REPS: _____
(Right Side)

→

2b. 4 Donkey Kicks to 4 High Knees

SET 1 REPS: _____

SET 2 REPS: _____

→

2c. Russian Twist

SET 1 REPS: _____

SET 2 REPS: _____

--- 30 SECOND BREAK ---

CIRCUIT 3

3a. 3-Point Lunge
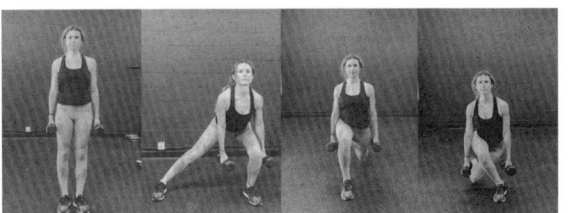

3b. In and Out Jack

(Left Side)	SET 1 REPS: _____	→	SET 1 REPS: _____
(Right Side)	SET 2 REPS: _____	→	SET 2 REPS: _____
(Alternate Sides)	SET 3 REPS: _____	→	SET 3 REPS: _____

--- 30 SECOND BREAK ---

CIRCUIT 4

4a. Burpee
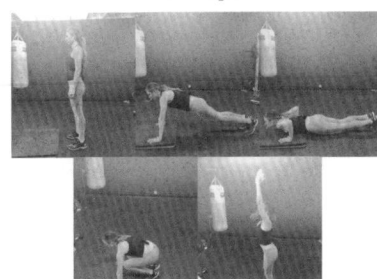

SET 1 REPS: _____ → 15s REST
SET 2 REPS: _____ → 15s REST
SET 3 REPS: _____ → 15s REST
SET 4 REPS: _____ → 15s REST

--- 30 SECOND BREAK ---

COOL DOWN

a. Butterfly Stretch

b. Runner's Stretch

c. Crossbody Hangover

d. Lat Stretch

HabitNest.link/booty15
EXERCISE GUIDE

Workout 15: Weight Training

DATE _____

1. Lateral Raise

SET 1	REPS: _____	(GOAL: 15-20)	WEIGHT: _____
SET 2	REPS: _____	(GOAL: 12-15)	WEIGHT: _____
SET 3	REPS: _____	(GOAL: 10-12)	WEIGHT: _____
SET 4 (Optional)	REPS: _____	(GOAL: 8-10)	WEIGHT: _____

2. Shoulder Rope Pull

SET 1	REPS: _____	(GOAL: 15-20)	WEIGHT: _____
SET 2	REPS: _____	(GOAL: 12-15)	WEIGHT: _____
SET 3	REPS: _____	(GOAL: 10-12)	WEIGHT: _____
SET 4 (Optional)	REPS: _____	(GOAL: 8-10)	WEIGHT: _____

3. Plank to Row

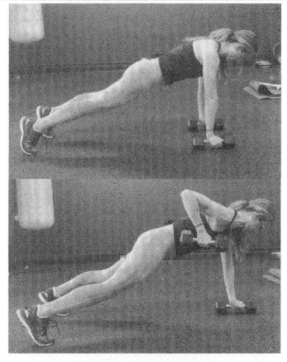

SET 1	REPS: _____	(GOAL: 15-20)	WEIGHT: _____
SET 2	REPS: _____	(GOAL: 12-15)	WEIGHT: _____
SET 3	REPS: _____	(GOAL: 10-12)	WEIGHT: _____
SET 4 (Optional)	REPS: _____	(GOAL: 8-10)	WEIGHT: _____

4. Deadlift

SET 1	REPS: _____	(GOAL: 15-20)	WEIGHT: _____
SET 2	REPS: _____	(GOAL: 12-15)	WEIGHT: _____
SET 3	REPS: _____	(GOAL: 10-12)	WEIGHT: _____
SET 4 (Optional)	REPS: _____	(GOAL: 8-10)	WEIGHT: _____

Workout 16: 4-3-2-1

HabitNest.link/booty16

DATE

GLUTE ACTIVATION WARMUP
30s EACH

a. Clam Opener

(30s Each Side)

b. Glute Bridge w/ Band Flutter

c. Fire Hydrant

(30s Each Leg)

d. Double Walk Out

(2 Steps Right, 2 Steps Left)

——————— 30 SECOND BREAK ———————

CIRCUIT 1
60s EACH

1a. Ski Mogul

REPS: _____ →

1b. Pendulum Lunge

REPS: _____
(Right Side) →

1c. Pendulum Lunge

REPS: _____
(Left Side) →

1d. Mountain Climber

REPS: _____
(Alternate Legs)

——————— 30 SECOND BREAK ———————

CIRCUIT 2
50s EACH

2a. 3-Point Lunge

(Left Side) SET 1 REPS: _____ →

(Right Side) SET 2 REPS: _____ →

2b. Side to Side Squat

SET 1 REPS: _____ →

SET 2 REPS: _____ →

2c. Side Shuffle w/ Floor Tap

SET 1 REPS: _____

SET 2 REPS: _____

---——— 30 SECOND BREAK ———---

 CIRCUIT 3

3a. Squat to Overhead Press

3b. Boxing Jab

SET 1 REPS: _____ → SET 1 REPS: _____

SET 2 REPS: _____ → SET 2 REPS: _____

SET 3 REPS: _____ → SET 3 REPS: _____

---——— 30 SECOND BREAK ———---

 CIRCUIT 4

4a. Jump Squat

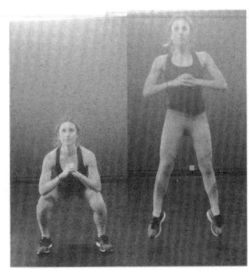

SET 1 REPS: _____ → 15s REST

SET 2 REPS: _____ → 15s REST

SET 3 REPS: _____ → 15s REST

SET 4 REPS: _____ → 15s REST

---——— 30 SECOND BREAK ———---

 COOL DOWN

a. Pigeon Stretch   b. Runner's Stretch   c. Crossbody Hangover   d. Hamstring Stretch

HabitNest.link/booty17
EXERCISE GUIDE

Workout 17: 4-3-2-1

DATE _____

 GLUTE ACTIVATION WARMUP

a. Clam Opener

(30s Each Side)

b. Glute Bridge w/ Band Flutter

c. Fire Hydrant

(30s Each Side)

d. Lateral Leg Raise

- 30s Each Leg (w/ Foot Flexed)
- 30s Each Leg (w/ Toes Pointing Down)

———————————— 30 SECOND BREAK ————————————

 ## CIRCUIT 1

1a. In and Out Jack

REPS: _____ →

1b. Leg Drop

REPS: _____ →

1c. High Knee

REPS: _____ →

1d. Russian Twist

REPS: _____

———————————— 30 SECOND BREAK ————————————

 ## CIRCUIT 2

2a. Plank Step Up

(Alternate Arms) SET 1 REPS: _____ →
(Alternate Arms) SET 2 REPS: _____ →

2b. Squat to Overhead Press

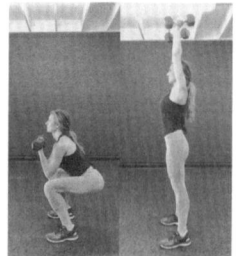

SET 1 REPS: _____ →
SET 2 REPS: _____ →

2c. Single Leg Glute Bridge

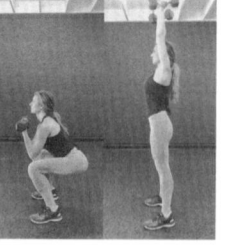

(Left Leg)   SET 1 REPS: _____
(Right Leg) SET 2 REPS: _____

─── 30 SECOND BREAK ───

CIRCUIT 3

3a. Side Plank w/ Torso Rotation   ### 3b. Ski Mogul

     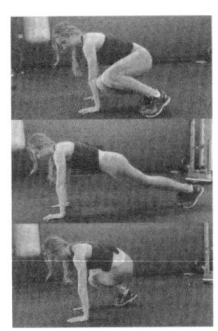

(Left Side)   SET 1 REPS: _____   →   SET 1 REPS: _____

(Right Side)   SET 2 REPS: _____   →   SET 2 REPS: _____

(Alternate Sides) SET 3 REPS: _____   →   SET 3 REPS: _____

─── 30 SECOND BREAK ───

CIRCUIT 4

4a. Burpee

SET 1 REPS: _____   →   15s REST

SET 2 REPS: _____   →   15s REST

SET 3 REPS: _____   →   15s REST

SET 4 REPS: _____   →   15s REST

─── 30 SECOND BREAK ───

COOL DOWN

a. Lat Stretch   **b. Glute Stretch**   **c. Pigeon Stretch**   **d. Runner's Stretch**

Workout 18: Weight Training

HabitNest.link/booty18

EXERCISE GUIDE

DATE _____

1. Squat

SET 1   REPS: _____   (GOAL: 15-20)   WEIGHT: _____
SET 2   REPS: _____   (GOAL: 12-15)   WEIGHT: _____
SET 3   REPS: _____   (GOAL: 10-12)   WEIGHT: _____
SET 4   REPS: _____   (GOAL: 8-10)   WEIGHT: _____
(Optional)

2. Alternating Step Up

SET 1   REPS: _____   (GOAL: 15-20)   WEIGHT: _____
SET 2   REPS: _____   (GOAL: 12-15)   WEIGHT: _____
SET 3   REPS: _____   (GOAL: 10-12)   WEIGHT: _____
SET 4   REPS: _____   (GOAL: 8-10)   WEIGHT: _____
(Optional)

3. Hip Thrust

SET 1   REPS: _____   (GOAL: 15-20)   WEIGHT: _____
SET 2   REPS: _____   (GOAL: 12-15)   WEIGHT: _____
SET 3   REPS: _____   (GOAL: 10-12)   WEIGHT: _____
SET 4   REPS: _____   (GOAL: 8-10)   WEIGHT: _____
(Optional)

4. Single Leg Deadlift

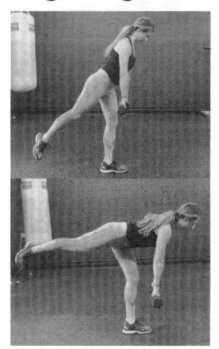

Left | Right

SET 1   REPS: _____   (GOAL: 15-20)   WEIGHT: _____
SET 2   REPS: _____   (GOAL: 12-15)   WEIGHT: _____
SET 3   REPS: _____   (GOAL: 10-12)   WEIGHT: _____
SET 4   REPS: _____   (GOAL: 8-10)   WEIGHT: _____
(Optional)

Workout 19: 4-3-2-1

HabitNest.link/booty19

EXERCISE GUIDE

DATE _____

 GLUTE ACTIVATION WARMUP
(30s EACH)

a. Clam Opener

(30s Each Side)

b. Tabletop w/Donkey Kick

c. Glute Bridge w/ Band Flutter

d. Lateral Leg Raise

- 30s Each Leg (w/ Foot Flexed)
- 30s Each Leg (w/ Toes Pointing Down)

---------- 30 SECOND BREAK ----------

 CIRCUIT 1
(60s EACH)

1a. Squat Thrust

1b. Side to Side Squat

1c. Fast Feet

1d. Side Triangle Crunch

REPS: _____ REPS: _____ → REPS: _____ → REPS: _____
(30s Each Side)

---------- 30 SECOND BREAK ----------

 CIRCUIT 2
(50s EACH)

2a. Side V-Up

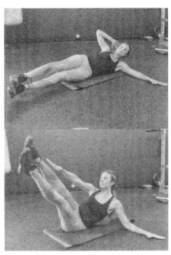

(Left Side) SET 1 REPS: _____
(Right Side) SET 2 REPS: _____

2b. Speed Skater

→ SET 1 REPS: _____
→ SET 2 REPS: _____

2c. Russian Twist

→ SET 1 REPS: _____
→ SET 2 REPS: _____

---------- 30 SECOND BREAK ----------

CIRCUIT 3

3a. 3-Point Lunge

3b. Burpee

(Left Leg)   SET 1 REPS: _____ → SET 1 REPS: _____

(Right Leg)   SET 2 REPS: _____ → SET 2 REPS: _____

(Alternate Legs) SET 3 REPS: _____ → SET 3 REPS: _____

---------- 30 SECOND BREAK ----------

CIRCUIT 4

4a. The Heisman

SET 1 REPS: _____ → 15s REST

SET 2 REPS: _____ → 15s REST

SET 3 REPS: _____ → 15s REST

SET 4 REPS: _____ → 15s REST

---------- 30 SECOND BREAK ----------

COOL DOWN

a. Pigeon Stretch   **b. Crossbody Hangover**   **c. Glute Stretch**   **d. Butterfly Stretch**

Workout 20: Weight Training

EXERCISE GUIDE — HabitNest.link/booty20

DATE: _____

1. Cable Row w/Squat

- **SET 1** REPS: _____ (GOAL: 15-20) WEIGHT: _____
- **SET 2** REPS: _____ (GOAL: 12-15) WEIGHT: _____
- **SET 3** REPS: _____ (GOAL: 10-12) WEIGHT: _____
- **SET 4** (Optional) REPS: _____ (GOAL: 8-10) WEIGHT: _____

2. Lat Pulldown

- **SET 1** REPS: _____ (GOAL: 15-20) WEIGHT: _____
- **SET 2** REPS: _____ (GOAL: 12-15) WEIGHT: _____
- **SET 3** REPS: _____ (GOAL: 10-12) WEIGHT: _____
- **SET 4** (Optional) REPS: _____ (GOAL: 8-10) WEIGHT: _____

3. Arnold Press

- **SET 1** REPS: _____ (GOAL: 15-20) WEIGHT: _____
- **SET 2** REPS: _____ (GOAL: 12-15) WEIGHT: _____
- **SET 3** REPS: _____ (GOAL: 10-12) WEIGHT: _____
- **SET 4** (Optional) REPS: _____ (GOAL: 8-10) WEIGHT: _____

4. Squat

- **SET 1** REPS: _____ (GOAL: 15-20) WEIGHT: _____
- **SET 2** REPS: _____ (GOAL: 12-15) WEIGHT: _____
- **SET 3** REPS: _____ (GOAL: 10-12) WEIGHT: _____
- **SET 4** (Optional) REPS: _____ (GOAL: 8-10) WEIGHT: _____

Check-In

How am I ACTUALLY feeling physically?

_____
_____
_____

How am I feeling about the quality and intensity of my workouts? Can I do more or am I pushing the limit consistently? Am I getting enough rest?

_____
_____
_____

How do I feel about the way I look? Do I see how much I can change if I stick to this program?

_____
_____
_____

What do I want to learn about this process that I can spend some time researching?

_____
_____
_____

Workout 21: 4-3-2-1

HabitNest.link/booty21

EXERCISE GUIDE

DATE

 GLUTE ACTIVATION WARMUP
(30s EACH)

a. Tabletop w/ Donkey Kick

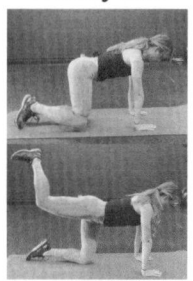

(30s Each Leg)

b. Box Draw

(Left Side)

c. Box Draw

(Right Side)

d. Tabletop w/ Diagonal Kick

(30s Each Leg)

——— 30 SECOND BREAK ———

 CIRCUIT 1
(60s EACH)

1a. Fast Feet

REPS: _____

→

1b. Lateral Lunge to Curtsy Lunge

REPS: _____
(Left Side)

→

1c. Lateral Lunge to Curtsy Lunge

REPS: _____
(Right Side)

→

1d. Speed Skater

REPS: _____

——— 30 SECOND BREAK ———

 CIRCUIT 2
(50s EACH)

2a. Plank Jack

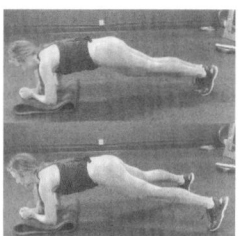

SET 1 REPS: _____

SET 2 REPS: _____

→

2b. Bulgarian Lunge

(Left Side) SET 1 REPS: _____

(Right Side) SET 2 REPS: _____

→

2c. Vertical Leap

SET 1 REPS: _____

SET 2 REPS: _____

─────────── 30 SECOND BREAK ───────────

CIRCUIT 3

3a. Woodchopper

3b. Roundhouse Kick to Squat

(Left Leg)   SET 1 REPS: _____   →   (Left Leg)   SET 1 REPS: _____
(Right Leg)   SET 2 REPS: _____   →   (Right Leg)   SET 2 REPS: _____
(Alternate Legs)   SET 3 REPS: _____   →   (Alternate Legs)   SET 3 REPS: _____

─────────── 30 SECOND BREAK ───────────

CIRCUIT 4

4a. Leap Forward in Squat, Burpee, & Shuffle Back

SET 1 REPS: _____   →   15s REST
SET 2 REPS: _____   →   15s REST
SET 3 REPS: _____   →   15s REST
SET 4 REPS: _____   →   15s REST

─────────── 30 SECOND BREAK ───────────

COOL DOWN

a. Hamstring Stretch   **b. Runner's Stretch**   **c. Pigeon Stretch**   **d. Crossbody Hangover**

Workout 22: 4-3-2-1

HabitNest.link/booty22

EXERCISE GUIDE

DATE _____

GLUTE ACTIVATION WARMUP 30s EACH

a. Tabletop w/ Donkey Kick

(30s Each Leg)

b. Box Draw

(Left Side)

c. Box Draw

(Right Side)

d. Running Man

(30s Each Side)

──────── 30 SECOND BREAK ────────

CIRCUIT 1 60s EACH

1a. Plank to Row

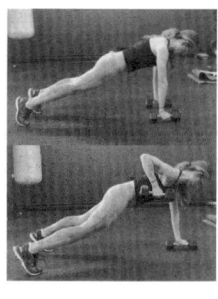

REPS: _____
(Alternate Arms)

→

1b. Leg Drop

REPS: _____

→

1c. Plie Squat w/ Shoulder Windmill

REPS: _____

→

1d. Spider-man Plank Crunch

REPS: _____
(Alternate Sides)

──────── 30 SECOND BREAK ────────

CIRCUIT 2 50s EACH

2a. 180° Jump Twist to Floor Tap

SET 1 REPS: _____

SET 2 REPS: _____

→

2b. Starfish Crunch

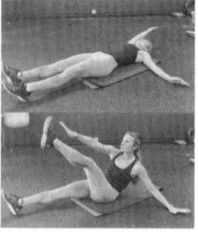

SET 1 REPS: _____
(Alternate Sides)

SET 2 REPS: _____
(Alternate Sides)

→

2c. Plank Step Up

SET 1 REPS: _____
(Alternate Arms)

SET 2 REPS: _____
(Alternate Arms)

─── 30 SECOND BREAK ───

CIRCUIT 3

3a. 4 Donkey Kicks to 4 High Knees

3b. Lateral Lunge w/ Knee to Elbow Rotation

SET 1 REPS: _____ → (Left Leg)   SET 1 REPS: _____

SET 2 REPS: _____ → (Right Leg)   SET 2 REPS: _____

SET 3 REPS: _____ → (Alternate Legs)   SET 3 REPS: _____

─── 30 SECOND BREAK ───

CIRCUIT 4

4a. Burpee

SET 1 REPS: _____ → 15s REST

SET 2 REPS: _____ → 15s REST

SET 3 REPS: _____ → 15s REST

SET 4 REPS: _____ → 15s REST

─── 30 SECOND BREAK ───

COOL DOWN

a. Lat Stretch

b. Glute Stretch

c. Pigeon Stretch

d. Butterfly Stretch

Workout 23: Weight Training

HabitNest.link/booty23

EXERCISE GUIDE

DATE _____

1. Deadlift

SET 1   REPS: _____   (GOAL: 15-20)   WEIGHT: _____
SET 2   REPS: _____   (GOAL: 12-15)   WEIGHT: _____
SET 3   REPS: _____   (GOAL: 10-12)   WEIGHT: _____
SET 4   REPS: _____   (GOAL: 8-10)   WEIGHT: _____
(Optional)

2. Squat

SET 1   REPS: _____   (GOAL: 15-20)   WEIGHT: _____
SET 2   REPS: _____   (GOAL: 12-15)   WEIGHT: _____
SET 3   REPS: _____   (GOAL: 10-12)   WEIGHT: _____
SET 4   REPS: _____   (GOAL: 8-10)   WEIGHT: _____
(Optional)

3. Single Leg Glute Bridge

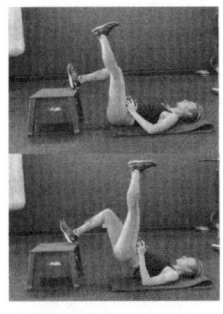

SET 1   REPS: _____   (GOAL: 15-20)   WEIGHT: _____
SET 2   REPS: _____   (GOAL: 12-15)   WEIGHT: _____
SET 3   REPS: _____   (GOAL: 10-12)   WEIGHT: _____
SET 4   REPS: _____   (GOAL: 8-10)   WEIGHT: _____
(Optional)

4. Alternating Step Up

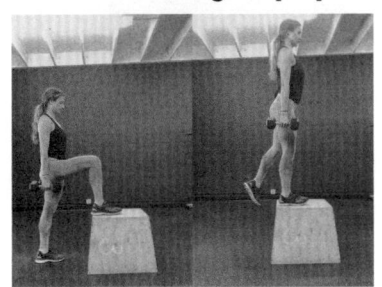

SET 1   REPS: _____   (GOAL: 15-20)   WEIGHT: _____
SET 2   REPS: _____   (GOAL: 12-15)   WEIGHT: _____
SET 3   REPS: _____   (GOAL: 10-12)   WEIGHT: _____
SET 4   REPS: _____   (GOAL: 8-10)   WEIGHT: _____
(Optional)

EXERCISE GUIDE — HabitNest.link/booty24

Workout 24: 4-3-2-1

DATE _____

 GLUTE ACTIVATION WARMUP (30s EACH)

a. Double Walk Out

(2 Steps Right, 2 Steps Left)

b. Box Draw

(Left Leg)

c. Box Draw

(Right Leg)

d. Tabletop w/ Diagonal Kick

(30s Each Leg)

———— 30 SECOND BREAK ————

 ## CIRCUIT 1 (60s EACH)

1a. Plank Jack

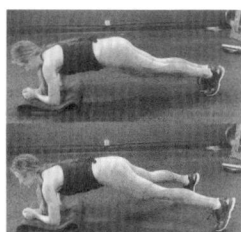

REPS: _____ →

1b. V-Up

REPS: _____ →

1c. Side Shuffle w/ Floor Tap

REPS: _____ →

1d. Lateral Lunge to Curtsy Lunge

REPS: _____
(30s Each Side)

———— 30 SECOND BREAK ————

 ## CIRCUIT 2 (50s EACH)

2a. Squat Thrust

SET 1 REPS: _____

SET 2 REPS: _____

→

2b. Tabletop Elbow to Knee Crunch

SET 1 REPS: _____
(Right Knee to Left Elbow)

SET 2 REPS: _____
(Right Knee to Left Elbow)

→

2c. Tabletop Elbow to Knee Crunch

SET 1 REPS: _____
(Left Knee to Right Elbow)

SET 2 REPS: _____
(Left Knee to Right Elbow)

─────────── 30 SECOND BREAK ───────────

 CIRCUIT 3

3a. Lateral Lunge w/ Half 'X'   3b. Mountain Climber

   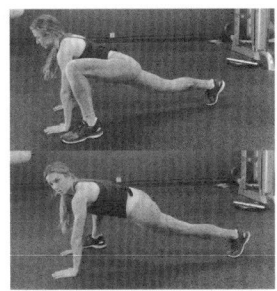

(Left Leg)   SET 1 REPS: _____   →   SET 1 REPS: _____
(Right Leg)   SET 2 REPS: _____   →   SET 2 REPS: _____
(Alternate Legs) SET 3 REPS: _____   →   SET 3 REPS: _____

─────────── 30 SECOND BREAK ───────────

 CIRCUIT 4

4a. Burpee

SET 1 REPS: _____   →   15s REST
SET 2 REPS: _____   →   15s REST
SET 3 REPS: _____   →   15s REST
SET 4 REPS: _____   →   15s REST

─────────── 30 SECOND BREAK ───────────

 COOL DOWN

a. Hamstring Stretch   **b. Butterfly Stretch**   **c. Glute Stretch**   **d. Crossbody Hangover**

Workout 25: Weight Training

HabitNest.link/booty25

EXERCISE GUIDE

DATE _____

1. Reverse Dumbbell Fly

SET 1	REPS: _____	(GOAL: 15-20)	WEIGHT: _____
SET 2	REPS: _____	(GOAL: 12-15)	WEIGHT: _____
SET 3	REPS: _____	(GOAL: 10-12)	WEIGHT: _____
SET 4 (Optional)	REPS: _____	(GOAL: 8-10)	WEIGHT: _____

2. Lat Pulldown

SET 1	REPS: _____	(GOAL: 15-20)	WEIGHT: _____
SET 2	REPS: _____	(GOAL: 12-15)	WEIGHT: _____
SET 3	REPS: _____	(GOAL: 10-12)	WEIGHT: _____
SET 4 (Optional)	REPS: _____	(GOAL: 8-10)	WEIGHT: _____

3. Arnold Press

SET 1	REPS: _____	(GOAL: 15-20)	WEIGHT: _____
SET 2	REPS: _____	(GOAL: 12-15)	WEIGHT: _____
SET 3	REPS: _____	(GOAL: 10-12)	WEIGHT: _____
SET 4 (Optional)	REPS: _____	(GOAL: 8-10)	WEIGHT: _____

4. Cable Row w/Squat

SET 1	REPS: _____	(GOAL: 15-20)	WEIGHT: _____
SET 2	REPS: _____	(GOAL: 12-15)	WEIGHT: _____
SET 3	REPS: _____	(GOAL: 10-12)	WEIGHT: _____
SET 4 (Optional)	REPS: _____	(GOAL: 8-10)	WEIGHT: _____

Workout 26: 4-3-2-1

HabitNest.link/booty26

EXERCISE GUIDE

DATE

 GLUTE ACTIVATION WARMUP (30s EACH)

a. Clam Opener

(30s Each Leg)

b. Glute Bridge w/ Leg Extension

(30s Each Leg)

c. Double Walk Out

(2 Steps Right, 2 Steps Left)

d. Lateral Leg Raise

- 30s Each Leg (w/ Foot Flexed)
- 30s Each Leg (w/ Toes Pointing Down)

──────────── 30 SECOND BREAK ────────────

 ## CIRCUIT 1 (60s EACH)

1a. Mountain Climber

REPS: _____
(Alternate Legs)

→

1b. 3-Point Lunge

REPS: _____
(Left Leg)

→

1c. 3-Point Lunge

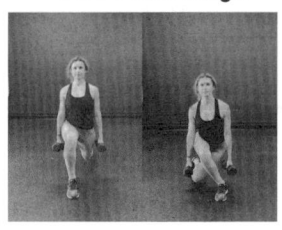

REPS: _____
(Right Leg)

→

1d. Boxing Jab

REPS: _____

──────────── 30 SECOND BREAK ────────────

 ## CIRCUIT 2 (50s EACH)

2a. The Heisman

SET 1 REPS: _____

SET 2 REPS: _____

→

2b. Pendulum Lunge

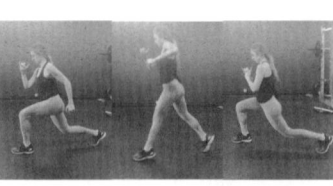

SET 1 REPS: _____

SET 2 REPS: _____

→

2c. Ski Mogul

SET 1 REPS: _____

SET 2 REPS: _____

─────────── 30 SECOND BREAK ───────────

 CIRCUIT 3
40s EACH

3a. Lateral Lunge to Curtsy Lunge   ### 3b. Side Shuffle w/ Floor Tap

          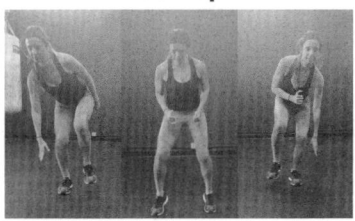

(Left Leg)   SET 1 REPS: _____   →   SET 1 REPS: _____
(Right Leg)   SET 2 REPS: _____   →   SET 2 REPS: _____
(Alternate Legs) SET 3 REPS: _____   →   SET 3 REPS: _____

─────────── 30 SECOND BREAK ───────────

 CIRCUIT 4
30s EACH

4a. Jump Squat

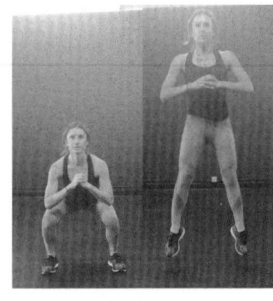

SET 1 REPS: _____   →   15s REST
SET 2 REPS: _____   →   15s REST
SET 3 REPS: _____   →   15s REST
SET 4 REPS: _____   →   15s REST

─────────── 30 SECOND BREAK ───────────

COOL DOWN
60s EACH

a. Hamstring Stretch   **b. Pigeon Stretch**   **c. Lat Stretch**   **d. Runner's Stretch**

         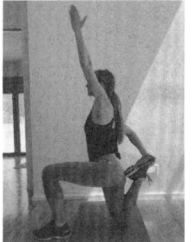

Workout 27: 4-3-2-1

HabitNest.link/booty27

EXERCISE GUIDE

DATE _____

GLUTE ACTIVATION WARMUP

30s EACH

a. Clam Opener

(30s Each Side)

b. Glute Bridge w/ Leg Extension

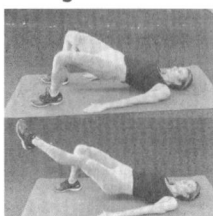

(Right Leg)

c. Glute Bridge w/ Leg Extension

(Right Leg)

d. Lateral Leg Raise

- 30s Each Leg (w/ Foot Flexed)
- 30s Each Leg (w/ Toes Pointing Down)

———————— 30 SECOND BREAK ————————

CIRCUIT 1

60s EACH

1a. Squat Thrust　　**1b. Standing Side Crunch**　　**1c. Standing Side Crunch**　　**1d. Plank to Row**

　　　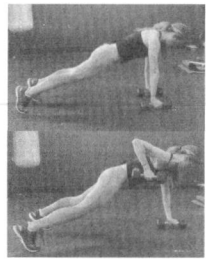

REPS: _____ → REPS: _____ → REPS: _____ → REPS: _____
　　　　　　　　　(Right Side)　　　　　(Left Side)

———————— 30 SECOND BREAK ————————

CIRCUIT 2

50s EACH

2a. Leg Drop　　　　**2b. Jump Twist**　　　　**2c. Russian Twist**

SET 1 REPS: _____ → SET 1 REPS: _____ → SET 1 REPS: _____

SET 2 REPS: _____ → SET 2 REPS: _____ → SET 2 REPS: _____

―――――― 30 SECOND BREAK ――――――

 ## CIRCUIT 3

3a. Squat to Overhead Press   3b. Starfish Crunch

     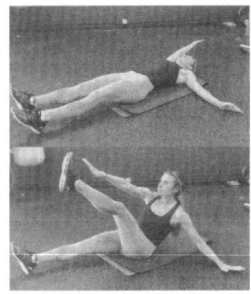

SET 1 REPS: _____   →   (Alternate Sides) SET 1 REPS: _____

SET 2 REPS: _____   →   (Alternate Sides) SET 2 REPS: _____

SET 3 REPS: _____   →   (Alternate Sides) SET 3 REPS: _____

―――――― 30 SECOND BREAK ――――――

 ## CIRCUIT 4

4a. 4 Donkey Kicks to 4 High Knees

SET 1 REPS: _____   →   REST

SET 2 REPS: _____   →   REST

SET 3 REPS: _____   →   REST

SET 4 REPS: _____   →   REST

―――――― 30 SECOND BREAK ――――――

 ## COOL DOWN

a. Glute Stretch   b. Pigeon Stretch   c. Hamstring Stretch   d. Butterfly Stretch

HabitNest.link/booty28

Workout 28: Weight Training

DATE _____

1. Hip Thrust

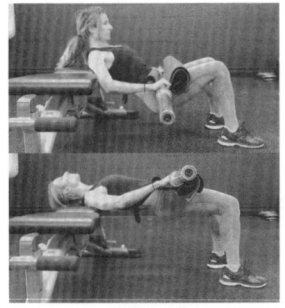

SET 1	REPS: _____	(GOAL: 15-20)	WEIGHT: _____
SET 2	REPS: _____	(GOAL: 12-15)	WEIGHT: _____
SET 3	REPS: _____	(GOAL: 10-12)	WEIGHT: _____
SET 4 (Optional)	REPS: _____	(GOAL: 8-10)	WEIGHT: _____

2. Squat

SET 1	REPS: _____	(GOAL: 15-20)	WEIGHT: _____
SET 2	REPS: _____	(GOAL: 12-15)	WEIGHT: _____
SET 3	REPS: _____	(GOAL: 10-12)	WEIGHT: _____
SET 4 (Optional)	REPS: _____	(GOAL: 8-10)	WEIGHT: _____

3. Elevated Plie Squat

SET 1	REPS: _____	(GOAL: 15-20)	WEIGHT: _____
SET 2	REPS: _____	(GOAL: 12-15)	WEIGHT: _____
SET 3	REPS: _____	(GOAL: 10-12)	WEIGHT: _____
SET 4 (Optional)	REPS: _____	(GOAL: 8-10)	WEIGHT: _____

4. Deadlift

SET 1	REPS: _____	(GOAL: 15-20)	WEIGHT: _____
SET 2	REPS: _____	(GOAL: 12-15)	WEIGHT: _____
SET 3	REPS: _____	(GOAL: 10-12)	WEIGHT: _____
SET 4 (Optional)	REPS: _____	(GOAL: 8-10)	WEIGHT: _____

Workout 29: 4-3-2-1

HabitNest.link/booty29

EXERCISE GUIDE

DATE

GLUTE ACTIVATION WARMUP

30s EACH

a. Clam Opener

(30s Each Side)

b. Tabletop w/ Donkey Kick

(30s Each Side)

c. Glute Bridge w/ Leg Extension

(30s Each Side)

d. Fire Hydrant

(30s Each Side)

--- 30 SECOND BREAK ---

CIRCUIT 1
60s EACH

1a. Leap Forward In Squat, Burpee, & Shuffle Back

REPS: _____ →

1b. Side Triangle Crunch

REPS: _____ (Left Side) →

1c. Side Triangle Crunch

REPS: _____ (Right Side) →

1d. Fast Feet

REPS: _____

--- 30 SECOND BREAK ---

CIRCUIT 2

50s EACH

2a. Roundhouse Kick to Squat

SET 1 REPS: _____ (Left Leg) →
SET 2 REPS: _____ (Right Leg) →

2b. Side Plank w/ Elbow Twist

SET 1 REPS: _____ (Right Side) →
SET 2 REPS: _____ (Left Side) →

2c. Ski Mogul

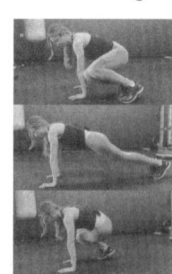

SET 1 REPS: _____
SET 2 REPS: _____

―――――――――――― 30 SECOND BREAK ――――――――――――

 ## CIRCUIT 3
40s EACH

3a. Lateral Lunge to Curtsy Lunge

3b. Starfish Crunch

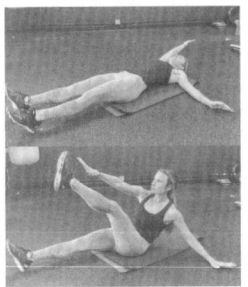

(Left Leg)	SET 1 REPS: _____	→	(Left Leg)	SET 1 REPS: _____
(Right Leg)	SET 2 REPS: _____	→	(Right Leg)	SET 2 REPS: _____
(Alternate Legs)	SET 3 REPS: _____	→	(Alternate Legs)	SET 3 REPS: _____

―――――――――――― 30 SECOND BREAK ――――――――――――

 ## CIRCUIT 4
30s EACH

4a. Burpee

SET 1 REPS: _____ → 15s REST
SET 2 REPS: _____ → 15s REST
SET 3 REPS: _____ → 15s REST
SET 4 REPS: _____ → 15s REST

―――――――――――― 30 SECOND BREAK ――――――――――――

 ## COOL DOWN
60s EACH

a. Pigeon Stretch

b. Glute Stretch

c. Hamstring Stretch

d. Crossbody Hangover

Workout 30: Weight Training

DATE _____

1. Deadlift

SET 1	REPS: _____	(GOAL: 15-20)	WEIGHT: _____
SET 2	REPS: _____	(GOAL: 12-15)	WEIGHT: _____
SET 3	REPS: _____	(GOAL: 10-12)	WEIGHT: _____
SET 4 (Optional)	REPS: _____	(GOAL: 8-10)	WEIGHT: _____

2. Shoulder Rope Pull

SET 1	REPS: _____	(GOAL: 15-20)	WEIGHT: _____
SET 2	REPS: _____	(GOAL: 12-15)	WEIGHT: _____
SET 3	REPS: _____	(GOAL: 10-12)	WEIGHT: _____
SET 4 (Optional)	REPS: _____	(GOAL: 8-10)	WEIGHT: _____

3. Lateral Raise

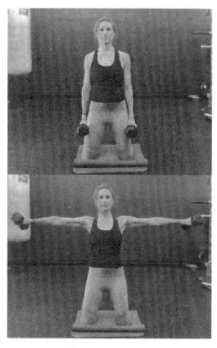

SET 1	REPS: _____	(GOAL: 15-20)	WEIGHT: _____
SET 2	REPS: _____	(GOAL: 12-15)	WEIGHT: _____
SET 3	REPS: _____	(GOAL: 10-12)	WEIGHT: _____
SET 4 (Optional)	REPS: _____	(GOAL: 8-10)	WEIGHT: _____

4. Hip Thrust

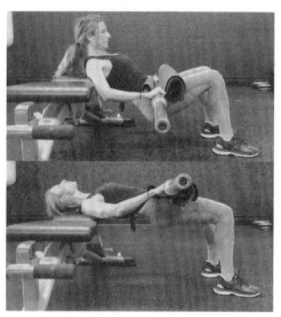

SET 1	REPS: _____	(GOAL: 15-20)	WEIGHT: _____
SET 2	REPS: _____	(GOAL: 12-15)	WEIGHT: _____
SET 3	REPS: _____	(GOAL: 10-12)	WEIGHT: _____
SET 4 (Optional)	REPS: _____	(GOAL: 8-10)	WEIGHT: _____

Check-In

How am I ACTUALLY feeling physically?

_____
_____
_____

How am I feeling about the quality and intensity of my workouts? Can I do more or am I pushing the limit consistently? Am I getting enough rest?

_____
_____
_____

How do I feel about the way I look? Do I see how much I can change if I stick to this program?

_____
_____
_____

What do I want to learn about this process that I can spend some time researching?

_____
_____
_____

Workout 31: 4-3-2-1

HabitNest.link/booty31

EXERCISE GUIDE

DATE _____

GLUTE ACTIVATION WARMUP
30s EACH

a. Double Walk Out

(2 Steps Right, 2 Steps Left)

b. Box Draw

(Right Leg)

c. Box Draw

(Left Leg)

d. Running Man

(30s Each Leg)

──── 30 SECOND BREAK ────

CIRCUIT 1
60s EACH

1a. Burpee

1b. Plie Squat w/ Shoulder Windmill

1c. Ski Mogul

1d. V-Up

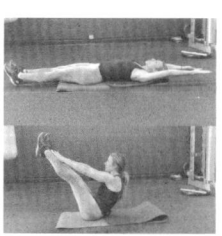

REPS: _____ → REPS: _____ → REPS: _____ → REPS: _____

──── 30 SECOND BREAK ────

CIRCUIT 2
50s EACH

2a. 4 Donkey Kicks to 4 High Knees

2b. Pendulum Jack

2c. Lateral Lunge to Curtsy Lunge

SET 1 REPS: _____ → SET 1 REPS: _____ → (Right Side) SET 1 REPS: _____

SET 2 REPS: _____ → SET 2 REPS: _____ → (Left Side) SET 2 REPS: _____

─── 30 SECOND BREAK ───

 ## CIRCUIT 3

3a. Plie Squat w/ Shoulder Windmill

3b. Jump Squat

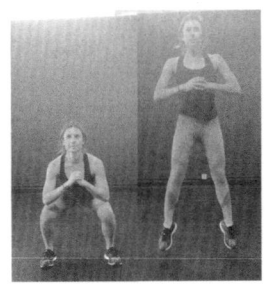

SET 1 REPS: _____ → SET 1 REPS: _____

SET 2 REPS: _____ → SET 2 REPS: _____

SET 3 REPS: _____ → SET 3 REPS: _____

─── 30 SECOND BREAK ───

 ## CIRCUIT 4

4a. In and Out Jack

SET 1 REPS: _____ → 15s REST

SET 2 REPS: _____ → 15s REST

SET 3 REPS: _____ → 15s REST

SET 4 REPS: _____ → 15s REST

─── 30 SECOND BREAK ───

 ## COOL DOWN

a. Runner's Stretch   b. Butterfly Stretch   c. Lat Stretch   d. Pigeon Stretch

HabitNest.link/booty32

Workout 32: 4-3-2-1

DATE _____

GLUTE ACTIVATION WARMUP
(30s EACH)

a. Double Walk Out

(2 Steps Right, 2 Steps Left)

b. Box Draw

(Left Leg)

c. Box Draw

(Right Leg)

d. Running Man

(30s Each Leg)

―――――――― 30 SECOND BREAK ――――――――

 ## CIRCUIT 1
(60s EACH)

1a. Boxing Jab

REPS: _____ →

1b. Plank Knee Tuck

REPS: _____
(Alternate Sides) →

1c. Vertical Sit-Up w/ Elbow to Knee Touch

REPS: _____
(Alternate Sides) →

1d. 180° Jump Twist to Floor Tap

REPS: _____

―――――――― 30 SECOND BREAK ――――――――

 ## CIRCUIT 2
(50s EACH)

2a. Leg Drop

SET 1 REPS: _____ →
SET 2 REPS: _____ →

2b. Squat Thrust

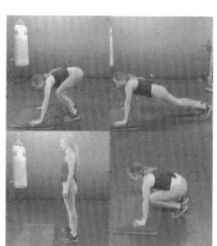

SET 1 REPS: _____ →
SET 2 REPS: _____ →

2c. Russian Twist

SET 1 REPS: _____
SET 2 REPS: _____

---------- 30 SECOND BREAK ----------

CIRCUIT 3

3a. Side Triangle Crunch   3b. Jump Squat

    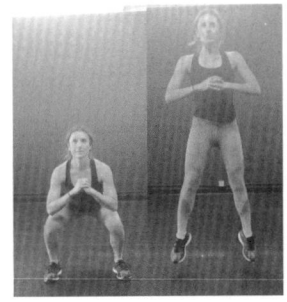

(Left Side)   SET 1 REPS: _____ → SET 1 REPS: _____

(Right Side)   SET 2 REPS: _____ → SET 2 REPS: _____

(Alternate Side) SET 3 REPS: _____ → SET 3 REPS: _____

---------- 30 SECOND BREAK ----------

CIRCUIT 4

4a. Burpee

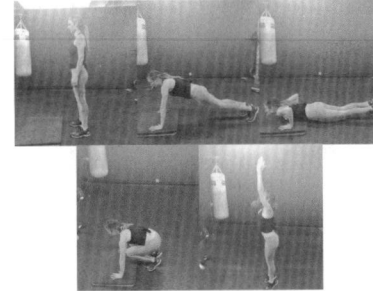

SET 1 REPS: _____ → 15s REST

SET 2 REPS: _____ → 15s REST

SET 3 REPS: _____ → 15s REST

SET 4 REPS: _____ → 15s REST

---------- 30 SECOND BREAK ----------

COOL DOWN

a. Butterfly Stretch   b. Hamstring Stretch   c. Lat Stretch   d. Glute Stretch

Workout 33: Weight Training

HabitNest.link/booty33

DATE _____

1. Deadlift

SET 1	REPS: _____	(GOAL: 15-20)	WEIGHT: _____
SET 2	REPS: _____	(GOAL: 12-15)	WEIGHT: _____
SET 3	REPS: _____	(GOAL: 10-12)	WEIGHT: _____
SET 4 (Optional)	REPS: _____	(GOAL: 8-10)	WEIGHT: _____

2. Squat

SET 1	REPS: _____	(GOAL: 15-20)	WEIGHT: _____
SET 2	REPS: _____	(GOAL: 12-15)	WEIGHT: _____
SET 3	REPS: _____	(GOAL: 10-12)	WEIGHT: _____
SET 4 (Optional)	REPS: _____	(GOAL: 8-10)	WEIGHT: _____

3. Hip Thrust

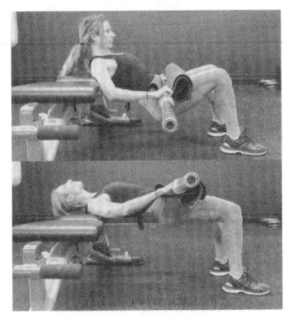

SET 1	REPS: _____	(GOAL: 15-20)	WEIGHT: _____
SET 2	REPS: _____	(GOAL: 12-15)	WEIGHT: _____
SET 3	REPS: _____	(GOAL: 10-12)	WEIGHT: _____
SET 4 (Optional)	REPS: _____	(GOAL: 8-10)	WEIGHT: _____

4. Woodchopper

	Left	Right		
SET 1	REPS: _____		(GOAL: 15-20)	WEIGHT: _____
SET 2	REPS: _____		(GOAL: 12-15)	WEIGHT: _____
SET 3	REPS: _____		(GOAL: 10-12)	WEIGHT: _____
SET 4 (Optional)	REPS: _____		(GOAL: 8-10)	WEIGHT: _____

Workout 34: 4-3-2-1

HabitNest.link/booty34
EXERCISE GUIDE

DATE

GLUTE ACTIVATION WARMUP

30s EACH

a. Tabletop w/ Diagonal Kick

(30s Each Leg)

b. Box Draw

(Right Leg)

c. Box Draw

(Left Leg)

d. Running Man

(30s Each Leg)

---- 30 SECOND BREAK ----

CIRCUIT 1

60s EACH

1a. Squat Thrust

REPS: _____ →

1b. V-Up

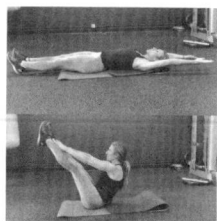

REPS: _____ →

1c. Side Shuffle w/ Floor Tap

REPS: _____ →

1d. Russian Twist

REPS: _____

---- 30 SECOND BREAK ----

CIRCUIT 2

50s EACH

2a. Lateral Lunge w/ Half-X

(Right Side) SET 1 REPS: _____ →
(Left Side) SET 2 REPS: _____ →

2b. Tabletop Elbow to Knee Crunch

SET 1 REPS: _____ →
(Right to Left)
SET 2 REPS: _____ →
(Left to Right)

2c. Speed Skater

SET 1 REPS: _____
SET 2 REPS: _____

---------- 30 SECOND BREAK ----------

CIRCUIT 3

3a. Lateral Lunge to Curtsy Lunge

3b. Side Plank w/ Torso Twist

(Left Side)   SET 1 REPS: _____   →   (Left Side)   SET 1 REPS: _____
(Right Side)   SET 2 REPS: _____   →   (Right Side)   SET 2 REPS: _____
(Alternate Sides)   SET 3 REPS: _____   →   (Alternate Sides)   SET 3 REPS: _____

---------- 30 SECOND BREAK ----------

CIRCUIT 4

4a. Jump Squat

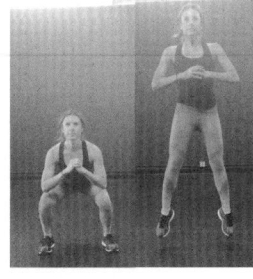

SET 1 REPS: _____ → 15s REST
SET 2 REPS: _____ → 15s REST
SET 3 REPS: _____ → 15s REST
SET 4 REPS: _____ → 15s REST

---------- 30 SECOND BREAK ----------

COOL DOWN

a. Hamstring Stretch   b. Pigeon Stretch   c. Runner's Stretch   d. Butterfly Stretch

Workout 35: Weight Training

DATE _____

1. Bent Over Row

SET 1 REPS: _____ (GOAL: 15-20) WEIGHT: _____
SET 2 REPS: _____ (GOAL: 12-15) WEIGHT: _____
SET 3 REPS: _____ (GOAL: 10-12) WEIGHT: _____
SET 4 REPS: _____ (GOAL: 8-10)   WEIGHT: _____
(Optional)

2. Reverse Dumbbell Fly

SET 1 REPS: _____ (GOAL: 15-20) WEIGHT: _____
SET 2 REPS: _____ (GOAL: 12-15) WEIGHT: _____
SET 3 REPS: _____ (GOAL: 10-12) WEIGHT: _____
SET 4 REPS: _____ (GOAL: 8-10)   WEIGHT: _____
(Optional)

3. Cable Row w/Squat

SET 1 REPS: _____ (GOAL: 15-20) WEIGHT: _____
SET 2 REPS: _____ (GOAL: 12-15) WEIGHT: _____
SET 3 REPS: _____ (GOAL: 10-12) WEIGHT: _____
SET 4 REPS: _____ (GOAL: 8-10)   WEIGHT: _____
(Optional)

4. Deadlift

SET 1 REPS: _____ (GOAL: 15-20) WEIGHT: _____
SET 2 REPS: _____ (GOAL: 12-15) WEIGHT: _____
SET 3 REPS: _____ (GOAL: 10-12) WEIGHT: _____
SET 4 REPS: _____ (GOAL: 8-10)   WEIGHT: _____
(Optional)

EXERCISE GUIDE: HabitNest.link/booty35

HabitNest.link/booty39

Workout 36: 4-3-2-1

DATE

GLUTE ACTIVATION WARMUP

a. Clam Opener

(30s Each Side)

b. Fire Hydrant

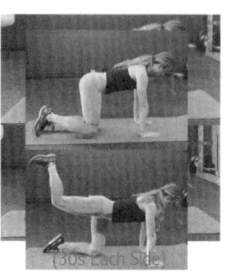

(30s Each Side)

c. Glute Bridge w/ Band Flutter

d. Double Walk Out

(2 Steps Right, 2 Steps Left)

───── 30 SECOND BREAK ─────

CIRCUIT 1

1a. Speed Skater

REPS: _____
(Alternate Sides)

1b. Pendulum Lunge

REPS: _____
(Left Leg)

1c. Pendulum Lunge

REPS: _____
(Right Leg)

1d. Mountain Climber

REPS: _____
(Alternate Sides)

───── 30 SECOND BREAK ─────

CIRCUIT 2

2a. Plie Squat w/ Shoulder Windmill

SET 1 REPS: _____

SET 2 REPS: _____

2b. Leap Forward in Squat, Burpee, & Shuffle Back

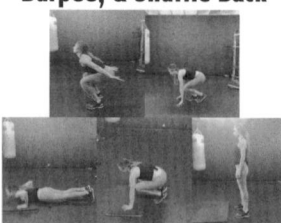

SET 1 REPS: _____

SET 2 REPS: _____

2c. Bulgarian Lunge

(Left Leg) SET 1 REPS: _____

(Right Leg) SET 2 REPS: _____

---——————————— 30 SECOND BREAK ———————————---

 CIRCUIT 3

3a. Vertical Leap

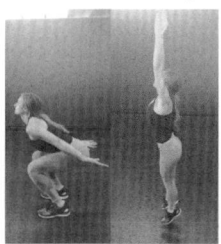

3b. Lateral Lunge w/ Knee to Elbow Rotation

SET 1 REPS: _____ → (Left Leg) SET 1 REPS: _____

SET 2 REPS: _____ → (Right Leg) SET 2 REPS: _____

SET 3 REPS: _____ → (Alternate Legs) SET 3 REPS: _____

---——————————— 30 SECOND BREAK ———————————---

 CIRCUIT 4

4a. Squat Jack

SET 1 REPS: _____ → 15s REST

SET 2 REPS: _____ → 15s REST

SET 3 REPS: _____ → 15s REST

SET 4 REPS: _____ → 15s REST

---——————————— 30 SECOND BREAK ———————————---

 COOL DOWN

a. Glute Stretch

b. Pigeon Stretch

c. Lat Stretch

d. Crossbody Hangover

HabitNest.link/booty37
EXERCISE GUIDE

Workout 37: 4-3-2-1

DATE _____

GLUTE ACTIVATION WARMUP
(30s EACH)

a. Clam Opener　　**b. Tabletop w/ Donkey Kick**　　**c. Glute Bridge w/ Band Flutter**　　**d. Lateral Leg Raise**

(30s Each Side)　　(30s Each Side)

- 30s Each Leg (w/ Foot Flexed)
- 30s Each Leg (w/ Toes Pointing Down)

────────── 30 SECOND BREAK ──────────

CIRCUIT 1
(60s EACH)

1a. Plank Jack　　**1b. Side Plank w/ Elbow Twist**　　**1c. Side Plank w/ Elbow Twist**　　**1d. Side Shuffle w/ Floor Tap**

REPS: _____ → REPS: _____ → REPS: _____ → REPS: _____
　　　　　　　　　　(Left Side)　　　　　(Right Side)

────────── 30 SECOND BREAK ──────────

CIRCUIT 2
(50s EACH)

2a. 3-Point Lunge　　**2b. Leg Drop**　　**2c. Mountain Climber**

(Left Leg) SET 1 REPS: _____ → SET 1 REPS: _____ → SET 1 REPS: _____

(Right Leg) SET 2 REPS: _____ → SET 2 REPS: _____ → SET 2 REPS: _____

──────── 30 SECOND BREAK ────────

 ## CIRCUIT 3

3a. Spider-man Plank Crunch   ### 3b. Side V-Up

(Alternate Sides)   SET 1 REPS: _____   →   (Left Side)   SET 1 REPS: _____
(Alternate Sides)   SET 2 REPS: _____   →   (Right Side)   SET 2 REPS: _____
(Alternate Sides)   SET 3 REPS: _____   →   (Alternate Sides) SET 3 REPS: _____

──────── 30 SECOND BREAK ────────

 ## CIRCUIT 4

4a. Burpee

SET 1 REPS: _____   →   15s REST
SET 2 REPS: _____   →   15s REST
SET 3 REPS: _____   →   15s REST
SET 4 REPS: _____   →   15s REST

──────── 30 SECOND BREAK ────────

 ## COOL DOWN

a. Crossbody Hangover   **b. Pigeon Stretch**   **c. Hamstring Stretch**   **d. Runner's Stretch**

Workout 38: Weight Training

HabitNest.link/booty38

DATE _____

1. Single Leg Glute Bridge

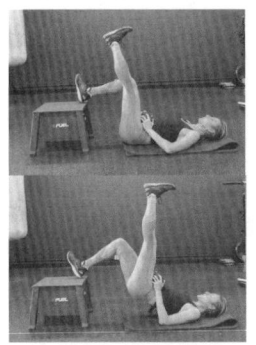

          Left   Right

SET 1   REPS: _____ (GOAL: 15-20)   WEIGHT: _____

SET 2   REPS: _____ (GOAL: 12-15)   WEIGHT: _____

SET 3   REPS: _____ (GOAL: 10-12)   WEIGHT: _____

SET 4   REPS: _____ (GOAL: 8-10)   WEIGHT: _____
(Optional)

2. Hip Thrusts

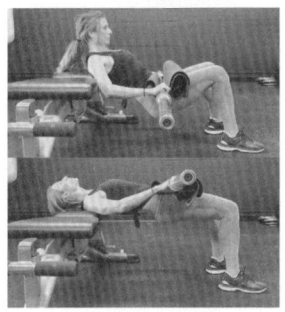

SET 1   REPS: _____ (GOAL: 15-20)   WEIGHT: _____

SET 2   REPS: _____ (GOAL: 12-15)   WEIGHT: _____

SET 3   REPS: _____ (GOAL: 10-12)   WEIGHT: _____

SET 4   REPS: _____ (GOAL: 8-10)   WEIGHT: _____
(Optional)

3. Alternating Step Up

SET 1   REPS: _____ (GOAL: 15-20)   WEIGHT: _____

SET 2   REPS: _____ (GOAL: 12-15)   WEIGHT: _____

SET 3   REPS: _____ (GOAL: 10-12)   WEIGHT: _____

SET 4   REPS: _____ (GOAL: 8-10)   WEIGHT: _____
Optional

4. Deadlift

SET 1   REPS: _____ (GOAL: 15-20)   WEIGHT: _____

SET 2   REPS: _____ (GOAL: 12-15)   WEIGHT: _____

SET 3   REPS: _____ (GOAL: 10-12)   WEIGHT: _____

SET 4   REPS: _____ (GOAL: 8-10)   WEIGHT: _____
(Optional)

EXERCISE GUIDE — HabitNest.link/booty39

Workout 39: 4-3-2-1

GLUTE ACTIVATION WARMUP (30s EACH)

a. Clam Opener   **b. Box Draw**   **c. Box Draw**   **d. Running Man**

(30s Each Side)

(Left Side)

(Right Side)

(30s Each Leg)

――― 30 SECOND BREAK ―――

CIRCUIT 1 (60s EACH)

1a. Bulgarian Lunge   **1b. Bulgarian Lunge**   **1c. Jump Twist**   **1d. Lateral Lunge**

REPS: _____ → REPS: _____ → REPS: _____ → REPS: _____
(Left Leg)   (Right Leg)   (Alternate Sides)

――― 30 SECOND BREAK ―――

CIRCUIT 2 (50s EACH)

2a. Squat Thrust   **2b. Squat to Overhead Press**   **2c. The Heisman**

SET 1 REPS: _____ → SET 1 REPS: _____ → SET 1 REPS: _____

SET 2 REPS: _____ → SET 2 REPS: _____ → SET 2 REPS: _____

----- 30 SECOND BREAK -----

CIRCUIT 3

3a. Spider-man Plank Crunch

3b. In and Out Jack

(Alternate Sides)	SET 1 REPS: _____	→	SET 1 REPS: _____
(Alternate Sides)	SET 2 REPS: _____	→	SET 2 REPS: _____
(Alternate Sides)	SET 3 REPS: _____	→	SET 3 REPS: _____

----- 30 SECOND BREAK -----

CIRCUIT 4

4a. Pendulum Jack

SET 1 REPS: _____ → 15s REST
SET 2 REPS: _____ → 15s REST
SET 3 REPS: _____ → 15s REST
SET 4 REPS: _____ → 15s REST

----- 30 SECOND BREAK -----

COOL DOWN

a. Hamstring Stretch

b. Glute Stretch

c. Butterfly Stretch

d. Pigeon Stretch

Workout 40: Weight Training

HabitNest.link/booty40

EXERCISE GUIDE

DATE _____

1. Lat Pulldown

SET 1	REPS: _____	(GOAL: 15-20)	WEIGHT: _____
SET 2	REPS: _____	(GOAL: 12-15)	WEIGHT: _____
SET 3	REPS: _____	(GOAL: 10-12)	WEIGHT: _____
SET 4 (Optional)	REPS: _____	(GOAL: 8-10)	WEIGHT: _____

2. Shoulder Rope Pull

SET 1	REPS: _____	(GOAL: 15-20)	WEIGHT: _____
SET 2	REPS: _____	(GOAL: 12-15)	WEIGHT: _____
SET 3	REPS: _____	(GOAL: 10-12)	WEIGHT: _____
SET 4 (Optional)	REPS: _____	(GOAL: 8-10)	WEIGHT: _____

3. Arnold Press

SET 1	REPS: _____	(GOAL: 15-20)	WEIGHT: _____
SET 2	REPS: _____	(GOAL: 12-15)	WEIGHT: _____
SET 3	REPS: _____	(GOAL: 10-12)	WEIGHT: _____
SET 4 (Optional)	REPS: _____	(GOAL: 8-10)	WEIGHT: _____

4. Squat

SET 1	REPS: _____	(GOAL: 15-20)	WEIGHT: _____
SET 2	REPS: _____	(GOAL: 12-15)	WEIGHT: _____
SET 3	REPS: _____	(GOAL: 10-12)	WEIGHT: _____
SET 4 (Optional)	REPS: _____	(GOAL: 8-10)	WEIGHT: _____

Check-In

How am I ACTUALLY feeling physically?

_____
_____
_____
_____

How am I feeling about the quality and intensity of my workouts? Can I do more or am I pushing the limit consistently? Am I getting enough rest?

_____
_____
_____
_____

How do I feel about the way I look? Do I see how much I can change if I stick to this program?

_____
_____
_____
_____

What do I want to learn about this process that I can spend some time researching?

_____
_____
_____
_____

Workout 41: 4-3-2-1

HabitNest.link/booty41

EXERCISE GUIDE

DATE _____

 GLUTE ACTIVATION WARMUP (30s EACH)

a. Double Walk Out

(2 Steps Right, 2 Steps Left)

b. Box Draw

(Left Leg)

c. Box Draw

(Right Leg)

d. Running Man

(30s Each Leg)

――― 30 SECOND BREAK ―――

 ## CIRCUIT 1 (60s EACH)

1a. Squat Jack

REPS: _____

1b. Plank to Row
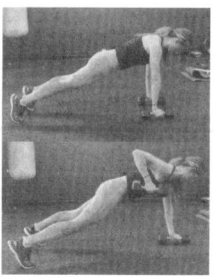
REPS: _____
(Alternate Arms)

1c. Plie Squat w/ Shoulder Windmill

REPS: _____

1d. Mountain Climber

REPS: _____
(Alternate Sides)

――― 30 SECOND BREAK ―――

 ## CIRCUIT 2 (50s EACH)

2a. 3-Point Lunge

(Left Leg) SET 1 REPS: _____
(Right Leg) SET 2 REPS: _____

2b. Side Triangle Crunch

(Left Side) SET 1 REPS: _____
(Right Side) SET 2 REPS: _____

2c. The Heisman

SET 1 REPS: _____
SET 2 REPS: _____

---30 SECOND BREAK---

 ## CIRCUIT 3

3a. Reverse Dumbbell Fly

3b. Leap Forward in Squat, Burpee, & Shuffle Back

SET 1 REPS: _____ → SET 1 REPS: _____

SET 2 REPS: _____ → SET 2 REPS: _____

SET 3 REPS: _____ → SET 3 REPS: _____

---30 SECOND BREAK---

 ## CIRCUIT 4

4a. 4 Donkey Kicks to 4 High Knees

SET 1 REPS: _____ → 15s REST

SET 2 REPS: _____ → 15s REST

SET 3 REPS: _____ → 15s REST

SET 4 REPS: _____ → 15s REST

---30 SECOND BREAK---

 ## COOL DOWN

a. Pigeon Stretch   b. Glute Stretch   c. Lat Stretch   d. Butterfly Stretch

Workout 42: 4-3-2-1

HabitNest.link/booty42

DATE

GLUTE ACTIVATION WARMUP
(30s EACH)

a. Double Walk Out

(2 Steps Right, 2 Steps Left)

b. Box Draw

(Left Leg)

c. Box Draw

(Right Leg)

d. Running Man

(30s Each Leg)

———————— 30 SECOND BREAK ————————

CIRCUIT 1
(60s EACH)

1a. Burpee

1b. Russian Twist

1c. Squat to Overhead Press

1d. Leg Drop

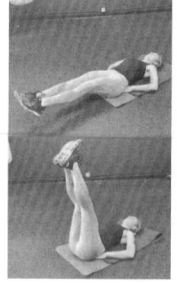

REPS: _____ → REPS: _____ → REPS: _____ → REPS: _____

———————— 30 SECOND BREAK ————————

CIRCUIT 2
(50s EACH)

2a. Plank Jack

2b. Side Triangle Crunch

2c. Mountain Climber

SET 1 REPS: _____ → (Left Side) SET 1 REPS: _____ → SET 1 REPS: _____

SET 2 REPS: _____ → (Right Side) SET 2 REPS: _____ → SET 2 REPS: _____

───── 30 SECOND BREAK ─────

 ## **CIRCUIT 3**

3a. Side Plank w/ Torso Rotation
3b. 180° Jump Twist to Floor Tap

(Left Leg)   SET 1 REPS: _____   →   SET 1 REPS: _____

(Right Leg)   SET 2 REPS: _____   →   SET 2 REPS: _____

(Alternate Legs)   SET t REPS: _____   →   SET 3 REPS: _____

───── 30 SECOND BREAK ─────

 ## **CIRCUIT 4**

4a. The Heisman

SET 1 REPS: _____   →   ⏱ REST

SET 2 REPS: _____   →   ⏱ REST

SET 3 REPS: _____   →   ⏱ REST

SET 4 REPS: _____   →   ⏱ REST

───── 30 SECOND BREAK ─────

 ## **COOL DOWN**

a. Pigeon Stretch   b. Lat Stretch   c. Butterfly Stretch   d. Runner's Stretch

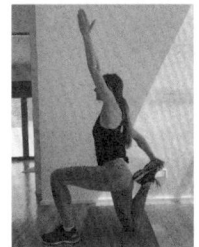

EXERCISE GUIDE
HabitNest.link/booty43

Workout 43: Weight Training

DATE _____

1. Deadlift

SET 1   REPS: _____   (GOAL: 15-20)   WEIGHT: _____
SET 2   REPS: _____   (GOAL: 12-15)   WEIGHT: _____
SET 3   REPS: _____   (GOAL: 10-12)   WEIGHT: _____
SET 4   REPS: _____   (GOAL: 8-10)   WEIGHT: _____
(Optional)

2. Squat

SET 1   REPS: _____   (GOAL: 15-20)   WEIGHT: _____
SET 2   REPS: _____   (GOAL: 12-15)   WEIGHT: _____
SET 3   REPS: _____   (GOAL: 10-12)   WEIGHT: _____
SET 4   REPS: _____   (GOAL: 8-10)   WEIGHT: _____
(Optional)

3. Hip Thrust

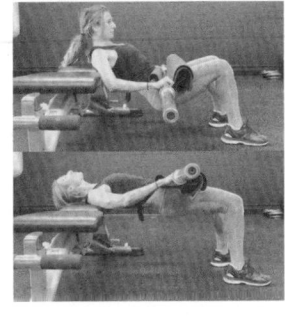

SET 1   REPS: _____   (GOAL: 15-20)   WEIGHT: _____
SET 2   REPS: _____   (GOAL: 12-15)   WEIGHT: _____
SET 3   REPS: _____   (GOAL: 10-12)   WEIGHT: _____
SET 4   REPS: _____   (GOAL: 8-10)   WEIGHT: _____
(Optional)

4. Single Leg Glute Bridge

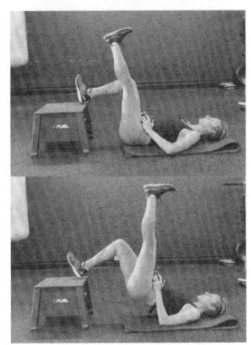

SET 1   REPS: _____   (GOAL: 15-20)   WEIGHT: _____
SET 2   REPS: _____   (GOAL: 12-15)   WEIGHT: _____
SET 3   REPS: _____   (GOAL: 10-12)   WEIGHT: _____
SET 4   REPS: _____   (GOAL: 8-10)   WEIGHT: _____
(Optional)

HabitNest.link/booty44
EXERCISE GUIDE

Workout 44: 4-3-2-1

DATE _____

GLUTE ACTIVATION WARMUP
(30s EACH)

a. Double Walk Out

(2 Steps Right, 2 Steps Left)

b. Tabletop w/ Donkey Kick

(30s Each Leg)

c. Tabletop w/ Diagonal Kick

(30s Each Leg)

d. Fire Hydrant

(30s Each Leg)

──────── 30 SECOND BREAK ────────

CIRCUIT 1
(60s EACH)

1a. Ski Mogul

1b. Lateral Lunge w/ Half 'X'

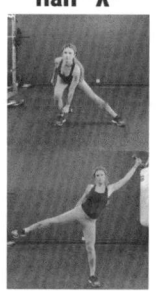

1c. Lateral Lunge w/ Half 'X'

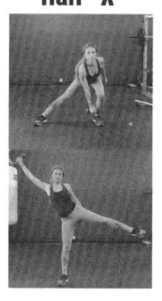

1d. Side Shuffle w/ Floor Tap

REPS: _____ → REPS: _____ → REPS: _____ → REPS: _____
                    (Left Leg)   (Right Leg)

──────── 30 SECOND BREAK ────────

CIRCUIT 2
(50s EACH)

2a. Squat Thrust

2b. Tabletop Elbow to Knee Crunch

2c. Jump Squat

SET 1 REPS: _____ → (Left Side) SET 1 REPS: _____ → SET 1 REPS: _____

SET 2 REPS: _____ → (Right Side) SET 2 REPS: _____ → SET 2 REPS: _____

─────────── 30 SECOND BREAK ───────────

 CIRCUIT 3
40s EACH

3a. Lateral Lunge to Curtsy Lunge   ### 3b. Side Triangle Crunch

(Left Leg)   SET 1 REPS: _____ →   SET 1 REPS: _____

(Right Leg)   SET 2 REPS: _____ →   SET 2 REPS: _____

(Alternate Legs) SET 3 REPS: _____ →   SET 3 REPS: _____

─────────── 30 SECOND BREAK ───────────

 CIRCUIT 4
30s EACH

4a. Burpee

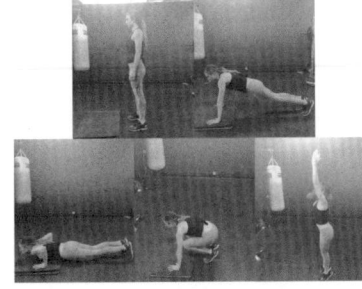

SET 1 REPS: _____ → 15s REST

SET 2 REPS: _____ → 15s REST

SET 3 REPS: _____ → 15s REST

SET 4 REPS: _____ → 15s REST

─────────── 30 SECOND BREAK ───────────

 COOL DOWN
60s EACH

a. Crossbody Hangover   **b. Runner's Stretch**   **c. Glute Stretch**   **d. Lat Stretch**

Workout 45: Weight Training

EXERCISE GUIDE — HabitNest.link/booty45

DATE _____

1. Reverse Dumbbell Fly

SET 1   REPS: _____   (GOAL: 15-20)   WEIGHT: _____
SET 2   REPS: _____   (GOAL: 12-15)   WEIGHT: _____
SET 3   REPS: _____   (GOAL: 10-12)   WEIGHT: _____
SET 4   REPS: _____   (GOAL: 8-10)   WEIGHT: _____
(Optional)

2. Shoulder Rope Pull

SET 1   REPS: _____   (GOAL: 15-20)   WEIGHT: _____
SET 2   REPS: _____   (GOAL: 12-15)   WEIGHT: _____
SET 3   REPS: _____   (GOAL: 10-12)   WEIGHT: _____
SET 4   REPS: _____   (GOAL: 8-10)   WEIGHT: _____
(Optional)

3. Bent Over Row

SET 1   REPS: _____   (GOAL: 15-20)   WEIGHT: _____
SET 2   REPS: _____   (GOAL: 12-15)   WEIGHT: _____
SET 3   REPS: _____   (GOAL: 10-12)   WEIGHT: _____
SET 4   REPS: _____   (GOAL: 8-10)   WEIGHT: _____
(Optional)

4. Lateral Raise

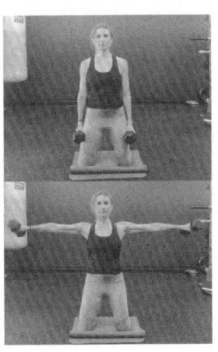

SET 1   REPS: _____   (GOAL: 15-20)   WEIGHT: _____
SET 2   REPS: _____   (GOAL: 12-15)   WEIGHT: _____
SET 3   REPS: _____   (GOAL: 10-12)   WEIGHT: _____
SET 4   REPS: _____   (GOAL: 8-10)   WEIGHT: _____
(Optional)

HabitNest.link/booty46
EXERCISE GUIDE

Workout 46: 4-3-2-1

DATE _____

GLUTE ACTIVATION WARMUP
30s EACH

a. Clam Opener   **b. Fire Hydrant**   **c. Tabletop w/ Donkey Kick**   **d. Double Walk Out**

      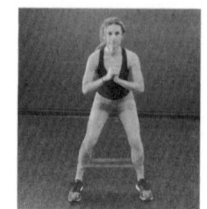

(30s Each Side)   (30s Each Side)   (30s Each Side)   (2 Steps Right, 2 Steps Left)

—— 30 SECOND BREAK ——

CIRCUIT 1
60s EACH

1a. In and Out Jack   **1b. Plie Squat w/ Shoulder Windmill**   **1c. High Knee**   **1d. Side to Side Squat**

REPS: _____ → REPS: _____ → REPS: _____ → REPS: _____
                                               (Alternate Sides)   (Alternate Sides)

—— 30 SECOND BREAK ——

CIRCUIT 2
50s EACH

2a. Speed Skater   **2b. Pendulum Lunge**   **2c. Fast Feet**

SET 1 REPS: _____ → (Left Leg) SET 1 REPS: _____ → SET 1 REPS: _____

SET 2 REPS: _____ → (Right Leg) SET 2 REPS: _____ → SET 2 REPS: _____

--- 30 SECOND BREAK ---

CIRCUIT 3

3a. Lateral Lunge to Curtsy Lunge   3b. Boxing Jab

(Left Leg)   SET 1 REPS: _____ → SET 1 REPS: _____

(Right Leg)   SET 2 REPS: _____ → SET 2 REPS: _____

(Alternate Legs) SET 3 REPS: _____ → SET 3 REPS: _____

--- 30 SECOND BREAK ---

CIRCUIT 4

4a. Burpee

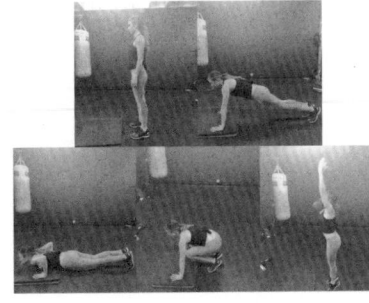

SET 1 REPS: _____ → 15s REST

SET 2 REPS: _____ → 15s REST

SET 3 REPS: _____ → 15s REST

SET 4 REPS: _____ → 15s REST

--- 30 SECOND BREAK ---

COOL DOWN

a. Hamstring Stretch   **b. Glute Stretch**   **c. Butterfly Stretch**   **d. Runner's Stretch**

   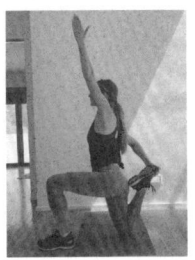

Workout 47: 4-3-2-1

HabitNest.link/booty47

EXERCISE GUIDE

DATE

GLUTE ACTIVATION WARMUP

30s EACH

a. Clam Opener

(30s Each Side)

b. Tabletop w/ Donkey Kick

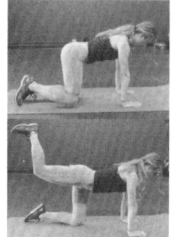

(30s Each Side)

c. Fire Hydrant

(30s Each Side)

d. Lateral Leg Raise

- 30s Each Leg (w/ Foot Flexed)
- 30s Each Leg (w/ Toes Pointing Down)

——————— 30 SECOND BREAK ———————

CIRCUIT 1

60s EACH

1a. Plank Step Up

REPS: _____
(Alternate Arms)

1b. Vertical Leap

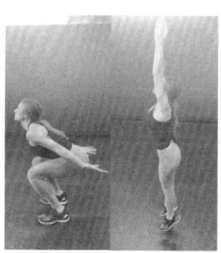

REPS: _____

1c. Side Triangle Crunch

REPS: _____
(Left Side)

1d. Side Triangle Crunch

REPS: _____
(Right Side)

——————— 30 SECOND BREAK ———————

CIRCUIT 2

50s EACH

2a. Squat Thrust

SET 1 REPS: _____

SET 2 REPS: _____

2b. V-Up

SET 1 REPS: _____

SET 2 REPS: _____

2c. Roundhouse Kick to Squat

(Left Leg) SET 1 REPS: _____

(Right Leg) SET 2 REPS: _____

---— 30 SECOND BREAK ———

CIRCUIT 3

3a. Lateral Lunge to Curtsy Lunge

3b. Mountain Climber

  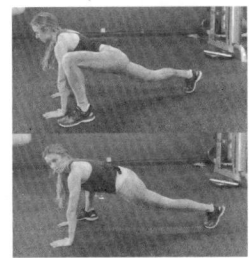

(Left Leg)	SET 1 REPS: _____	→	SET 1 REPS: _____
(Right Leg)	SET 2 REPS: _____	→	SET 2 REPS: _____
(Alternate Legs)	SET 3 REPS: _____	→	SET 3 REPS: _____

——— 30 SECOND BREAK ———

CIRCUIT 4

4a. Burpee

SET 1 REPS: _____ → 15s REST
SET 2 REPS: _____ → 15s REST
SET 3 REPS: _____ → 15s REST
SET 4 REPS: _____ → 15s REST

——— 30 SECOND BREAK ———

COOL DOWN

a. Hamstring Stretch   b. Crossbody Hangover   c. Pigeon Stretch   d. Butterfly Stretch

Workout 48: Weight Training

HabitNest.link/booty48

EXERCISE GUIDE

DATE _____

1. Single Leg Glute Bridge

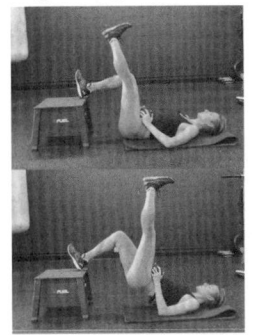

		Left	Right		
SET 1	REPS: _____			(GOAL: 15-20)	WEIGHT: _____
SET 2	REPS: _____			(GOAL: 12-15)	WEIGHT: _____
SET 3	REPS: _____			(GOAL: 10-12)	WEIGHT: _____
SET 4 (Optional)	REPS: _____			(GOAL: 8-10)	WEIGHT: _____

2. Hip Thrust

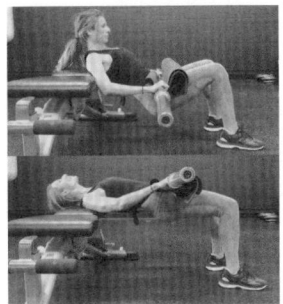

SET 1	REPS: _____	(GOAL: 15-20)	WEIGHT: _____
SET 2	REPS: _____	(GOAL: 12-15)	WEIGHT: _____
SET 3	REPS: _____	(GOAL: 10-12)	WEIGHT: _____
SET 4 (Optional)	REPS: _____	(GOAL: 8-10)	WEIGHT: _____

3. Single Leg Deadlift

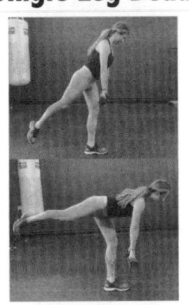

		Left	Right		
SET 1	REPS: _____			(GOAL: 15-20)	WEIGHT: _____
SET 2	REPS: _____			(GOAL: 12-15)	WEIGHT: _____
SET 3	REPS: _____			(GOAL: 10-12)	WEIGHT: _____
SET 4 (Optional)	REPS: _____			(GOAL: 8-10)	WEIGHT: _____

4. Squat

SET 1	REPS: _____	(GOAL: 15-20)	WEIGHT: _____
SET 2	REPS: _____	(GOAL: 12-15)	WEIGHT: _____
SET 3	REPS: _____	(GOAL: 10-12)	WEIGHT: _____
SET 4 (Optional)	REPS: _____	(GOAL: 8-10)	WEIGHT: _____

HabitNest.link/booty49
EXERCISE GUIDE

Workout 49: 4-3-2-1

DATE _____

GLUTE ACTIVATION WARMUP
(30s EACH)

a. Double Walk Out

(2 Steps Right, 2 Steps Left)

b. Box Draw

(Right Leg)

c. Box Draw

(Left Leg)

d. Running Man

(30s Each Leg)

──── 30 SECOND BREAK ────

 ## CIRCUIT 1
(60s EACH)

1a. In and Out Jack

REPS: _____ →

1b. Plank to Row

REPS: _____ →
(Alternate Arms)

1c. Mountain Climber

REPS: _____ →
(Alternate Sides)

1d. Starfish Crunch

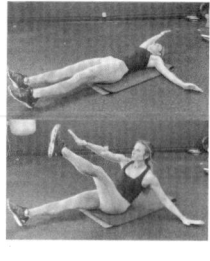

REPS: _____
(Alternate Sides)

──── 30 SECOND BREAK ────

 ## CIRCUIT 2
(50s EACH)

2a. Roundhouse Kick to Squat

(Left Leg) SET 1 REPS: _____ →

(Right Leg) SET 2 REPS: _____ →

2b. Side Plank w/ Torso Rotation

(Left Side) SET 1 REPS: _____ →

(Right Side) SET 2 REPS: _____ →

2c. The Heisman

SET 1 REPS: _____

SET 2 REPS: _____

―― 30 SECOND BREAK ――

CIRCUIT 3

3a. Plie Jump Squat

3b. Standing Side Crunch

SET 1 REPS: _____   → (Left Side)   SET 1 REPS: _____

SET 2 REPS: _____   → (Right Side)   SET 2 REPS: _____

SET 3 REPS: _____   → (Alternating Sides) SET 3 REPS: _____

―― 30 SECOND BREAK ――

CIRCUIT 4

4a. Leap Forward in Squat, Burpee, & Shuffle Back

SET 1 REPS: _____ → 15s REST

SET 2 REPS: _____ → 15s REST

SET 3 REPS: _____ → 15s REST

SET 4 REPS: _____ → 15s REST

―― 30 SECOND BREAK ――

COOL DOWN

a. Pigeon Stretch   **b. Runner's Stretch**   **c. Glute Stretch**   **d. Lat Stretch**

Workout 50: Weight Training

DATE _____

1. Squat

SET 1	REPS: _____	(GOAL: 15-20)	WEIGHT: _____
SET 2	REPS: _____	(GOAL: 12-15)	WEIGHT: _____
SET 3	REPS: _____	(GOAL: 10-12)	WEIGHT: _____
SET 4 (Optional)	REPS: _____	(GOAL: 8-10)	WEIGHT: _____

2. Reverse Dumbbell Fly

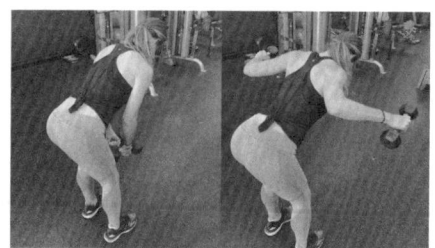

SET 1	REPS: _____	(GOAL: 15-20)	WEIGHT: _____
SET 2	REPS: _____	(GOAL: 12-15)	WEIGHT: _____
SET 3	REPS: _____	(GOAL: 10-12)	WEIGHT: _____
SET 4 (Optional)	REPS: _____	(GOAL: 8-10)	WEIGHT: _____

3. Lat Pulldown

SET 1	REPS: _____	(GOAL: 15-20)	WEIGHT: _____
SET 2	REPS: _____	(GOAL: 12-15)	WEIGHT: _____
SET 3	REPS: _____	(GOAL: 10-12)	WEIGHT: _____
SET 4 (Optional)	REPS: _____	(GOAL: 8-10)	WEIGHT: _____

4. Lateral Raise

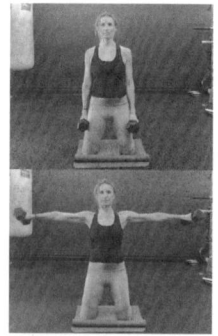

SET 1	REPS: _____	(GOAL: 15-20)	WEIGHT: _____
SET 2	REPS: _____	(GOAL: 12-15)	WEIGHT: _____
SET 3	REPS: _____	(GOAL: 10-12)	WEIGHT: _____
SET 4 (Optional)	REPS: _____	(GOAL: 8-10)	WEIGHT: _____

EXERCISE GUIDE: HabitNest.link/booty50

Congratulations!!!

You've made it to the end of the journal and completed an INTENSE interval training & weightlifting regimen that has no doubt increased your strength, appearance, confidence, and ability to accomplish your goals.

For you to have gotten this far means you've earned a very serious congratulations. You need to celebrate because your willpower and confidence should be soaring through the roof.

You've gained lessons about yourself not many dare to approach. You've struggled with your own mind, body and heart and gained some serious control over them. You fully understand that you have the power in you to accomplish ANY goal you put your mind to.

That's so awesome.

You are a true WARRIOR.

Note: We constantly (daily!) read reviews for all of our products on Amazon. It would mean the absolute world if you could leave us a genuine review of the journal there.

And if for any reason you had any issues with the journal, please email us directly at smile@habitnest.com so we can take care of you.

Check-In

How has my life changed since I started this program?

_____
_____
_____
_____

What changes have I seen in my attitude?

_____
_____
_____
_____

What physical changes have I seen?

_____
_____
_____
_____

How do I feel about myself in general compared to when I started this program?

_____
_____
_____
_____

How do I see myself continuing to build on what I've learned and gained by doing this program?

_____
_____
_____
_____

- Fin -

So, What Now?

So you've gotten through the program, seen incredible results, learned that you have immense strength in you to accomplish your goals, and hopefully you're more confident than ever!

Although you should feel very accomplished for getting through this entire program… know that you started the program to continually improve your life. *Don't stop now. This is only the beginning.*

Remember: **Every single day in your life where you take the time to work towards a more physically energized, fitter, confident version of yourself will automatically be a better day in your life.**

You only stand to gain from continuing work towards your fitness goals.

About the Authors

Amir Atighehchi graduated from USC's Marshall School of Business in 2013. He began to study the behaviors of the world's most successful people. This catapulted him to start building many "success-habits" into his daily routine. He's a big believer in BJ Fogg's Tiny Habits™ model and applies it to every new habit he forms. Mikey and Amir are also co-founders of the bicycle lock company, Nutlock.

Mikey Ahdoot transformed his life from a 200+ pound, video game addict to someone who was doing 17 daily habits consistently at one point. From ice cold showers to brainstorming 10 ideas a day (shoutout to James Altucher) to celebrating life every damn day, he first hand is becoming a habit routine machine that sets himself up for success daily. He is a graduate of USC's Marshall School of Business and proud trojan.

Ariel Banayan began studying habits and their relation to success when he was seventeen. Through experimenting with different lifestyle habits, he quickly learned how important it is to take care of ourselves mentally, physically and emotionally to operate at maximum capacity. Ariel graduated at the top of his class from the University of Southern California Gould School of Law in 2016.

Jennifer Cohen is a best-selling author, consultant, entrepreneur, fitness and health expert. Her stellar reputation has been built on a savvy, straight-talking approach and belief in a "no excuse" approach that forgoes the fads and focuses on long-term, sustainable results.
Jen has been a spokesperson and consultant for brands like Weight Watchers, KIND Bars and Muscle Milk. She has been named in "Greatest" 100 most influential people in Health and Fitness" and #16 Most Impactful Fitness Entrepreneurs on Web MD. Jennifer is also a loving wife and a mother to two children.

Shop Jen Cohen / Habit Nest Products

Strong Is The New Skinny
by Jennifer Cohen

Sick and tired of hearing what's wrong with you and your body? You're not alone.

It's time for a new conversation—and a new plan for treating, feeding, and moving your body in ways that build on your strengths inside and out.

Strong is sexy. Strong is powerful. Strong is achievable.

With STRONG IS THE NEW SKINNY you can say goodbye to body-bashing and physical faultfinding, and instead learn to embrace, not just how it looks, but what your body can do—from pushups to pull ups and box jumps to rope climbs, nothing is out of your reach.

Strong Is the New Skinny offers a reality-based diet, lifestyle, and fitness program (the "SINS" plan, for short) so you can:

- Maximize your potential, as well as your energy, vitality, and power.

- Train your brain—develop resilience and mental fortitude in every area of your life.

- Add muscle, increase speed, and enhance flexibility.

- Strengthen your arms, back, core, and legs—and crank up the challenge when you're ready for the next level.

- Torch fat with Strong Moves: a series of heart-healthy H.I.I.T. workouts that take as little as 10 minutes.

- Kick-start your Get-Fit, Get-Fierce plan with the Strong Seven—7 days of 7 power foods.

Whether you're just getting started or training for a challenging physical event, this book gives you all the tools you need to become leaner, fitter, and stronger: nutritionally, physically, psychologically, and emotionally.

Morning Sidekick Journal

The *Morning Sidekick Journal* is the first journal we created at Habit Nest. It begins by walking through the What, the How, and the Why of building morning routines with an intro section (~35 pages), followed by 66 days of content and 66 days of tracking to help instill the habit within you.

Morning routines are shown to be one of the most **critical elements of winning your day**. Starting your day off on the right foot sets the tone for the rest of it.

The journal is specifically designed to **create a cycle of accountability** within yourself by using your nights to hold you accountable in the morning, and your mornings to map out what's needed for that night.

It's jam-packed with effective and actionable content that will help you build this habit in bite sized chunks.

Like all of our products, the Morning Sidekick Journal comes with a 50 year satisfaction guarantee.

One thing we love: Regardless of what time you wake up, the journal will show you how to create a routine (short or long) that works for you.

Get yours at: SidekickJournal.com/morning

Sample Journal Page

_____
DATE

Night 0

(Begin Nighttime Routine).

TONIGHT I'LL SLEEP AT: **11:30pm** & TOMORROW I'LL WAKE UP AT: **6:30am**

🪄 MAGICAL MOMENT(S) I EXPERIENCED TODAY:

Watching the sunrise on my morning run :)

Finally made progress on my side-business!

☀ MY MORNING RITUAL TOMORROW WILL BE:

Completed?

1. 5 minutes of meditation ✓
2. Read 2 pages of "Think and Grow Rich" ✓
3. Affirmations ☐
4. Walk 2 blocks outside ☐
5. Plan out and strategize the rest of my day ☐

Day 1

(Begin Morning Routine).

LAST NIGHT I SLEPT AT: **12am** & WOKE UP TODAY AT: **7am**

🐎 MY MOST IMPORTANT TASK FOR TODAY IS:

Begin designing the app for my new startup

⊕ ONE WAY I CAN IMPROVE LIFE BY 1% IS:

Less Facebook / Instagram in the mornings

🧘 TOP TWO DISTRACTIONS TO MINIMIZE TONIGHT (BEFORE BED):

1. Watching YouTube in bed (limit: 15mins)
2. Watching the news (limit: 15mins)

Nutrition & Weight Management Sidekick
Journal

The *Nutrition & Weight Management Sidekick Journal* makes for a fantastic companion to fitness and exercise goals.

It's designed to be flexible and adaptable to whatever food goals you may have. Users have successfully used it to implement:

- Calorie counting
- Fat loss and/or muscle building
- General healthy eating
- Paleo / vegan / IIFYM / ketosis / other custom diets

The journal serves as your personal trainer for losing weight and **regaining control over your eating habits** quickly and effectively.

It allows you to **perfectly track** all that you need for YOUR body's optimum nutrition and fat loss. These include:

- Daily caloric intake goal
- Water drinking goal
- Exercise goal
- Planned vs. actual meals, (& caloric intake for each)
- Snacks, alcohol, and other intake
- Upcoming big meals to watch out for

One thing we love: A lot of the tips are designed to help you **break the association** that may exist between **your confidence / happiness** and **your body weight.**

Get yours at SidekickJournal.com/nutrition

Sample Journal Page

TODAY'S CALORIE GOAL   DATE

A 100-200 calorie range works well!   1,900 – 2,100 ☑

WATER DRINKING GOAL   **EXERCISE GOAL**

Two 500mL bottles ☑   2 mile jog ☐

TODAY'S MEALS

(Optional)

	Planned	Actual	Calories Eaten?
1.	3 eggs w/ 2 rice cakes	3 eggs w/ 2 rice cakes	340
2.	Chicken + Broccoli + cauliflower	Burrito (tortilla, avocado, tomatoes, chicken)	800
3.	Salmon w/ asparagus	Salmon w/ asparagus	500
4.			
5.			

SNACKS, DRINKS, & OTHER

30 almonds	210
One snickerdoodle cookie	250

TODAY'S TOTAL: **2,100**

POTENTIAL FOOD OBSTACLE(S) TO LOOK OUT FOR TOMORROW:

Resist the cookies at lunch!

ONE WAY I CAN IMPROVE BY 1% TOMORROW IS:

If I bring a snack to work, I can eat that instead of sweets.

Meditation Sidekick
Journal

This journal is built to help two types of people:

1. To help **newcomers or past strugglers** to easily own the practice of meditation.

2. To help **constant meditators** push their practice to another level.

Layout of the journal

1. **Building the foundation** - get a quick insight into the *science behind meditation* and get an idea of what you're likely to experience during it.

2. **Accountability** - track your practice daily to see your progress and hold yourself accountable in staying consistent.

3. **Learn in bite-sized chunks** - get daily exposure to different types of meditations (i.e. transcendental, gratitude, physical body, etc.) and see which ones impact your life the most.

One thing we love: The journal is not just designed to help you meditate effectively, but more importantly, to **help you reach the end goal of consistently living mindfully every day.**

Get yours at SidekickJournal.com/meditation

Sample Journal Page

DATE _____

TODAY I WILL MEDITATE AT: 7:30 a.m. ✓

FOR AT LEAST: 5 minutes ✓

ONE UPCOMING MENTAL OR EMOTIONAL HURDLE TO BE MINDFUL OF:

My presentation for my boss at work – own it!

BENEFITS I FELT TODAY (CIRCLE):

Feel Happier · More Creative · Increased Willpower · Improved Focus · More Energized · Reduced Stress

WHAT DOES MY INTERNAL DIALOGUE CONSIST OF?

I realize that I think about my appearance A LOT... and I immediately assume people judge me for it.

ONE SMALL WAY I CAN IMPROVE MY INTERNAL DIALOGUE:

I could be more understanding when I'm feeling self-conscious and willingly accept myself for how I look.

OPENING UP ABOUT MY DAY:

Today was a rollercoaster. I realize that when I'm working with others, I prefer not to rely on them to get things done. It's something I want to work on improving because I make myself feel anxious when it happens.

The Greatest Gift

The Greatest Gift helps you build the incredible habit of gratitude… and give a gift of pure love at the same time.

It's a gratitude journal you fill out with 21 stories for **one specific person** of how they've impacted your life and how you're thankful for them.

When you're finished, you **surprise them** with the finished journal as a gift.

We help you tell your story with:
- **30 story ideas** to spark what to write about
- **Specific guidance** on how to tell your story
- Journal + box + card + envelope + ribbon + wrapping paper to make the **perfect presentation they'll remember FOREVER**

Skyrocket your positivity and appreciation for the world, all while giving a heartfelt gift of gratitude to someone you love.

Get yours at: **greatestgift.io**

Share The Love

If you're reading this, that means you've come pretty far from where you were a couple months ago. You should be extremely proud of yourself!

If you believe this journal has had a positive impact on your life, we invite you to consider gifting a new one to a friend.

Is there a holiday coming up? Is there a special birthday around the corner? Or do you just want to put a smile on someone's face and do something incredible for them?

Gifting this journal is the absolute best way to show any gratitude you may have for what we've written here, as well as serving as a force of good through giving back to others. And you can rest assured that you're helping improve another person's life at the same time.

If you decide to, feel free to re-order here: www.HabitNest.com

Workout Index

1. Glute Activation Warmups
2. 4-3-2-1 Leg and Cardio Exercises
3. Weight Training Strength Exercises
4. 4-3-2-1 Waist Exercises
5. Weight Training Shoulder & Back Exercises
6. Stretches

Glute Activation Warmups

4 Donkey Kicks to 4 High Knees

1. Start in a downward dog position with your arms and fee shoulder-width apart.

2. Kick your feet and calves upwards towards your tailbone while bracing your core and shifting your weight to your arms.

3. Repeat this three more times.

4. Stand straight up with your feet shoulder-width apart.

5. Run in place 4 times while raising your knees as high as possible as you alternate legs.

6. Repeat until the set is complete!

Glute Activation Warmups

Box Draw

1. Wrap the resistance band around your calves or ankles.

2. Get into a squat position with your knees bent and your feet shoulder-width apart.

3. Staying low in squat position, take a step forward, then to the right, then behind you, and then diagonally behind you all with the same leg.

4. Keep your core tight and your glute muscles squeezed as you complete the exercise.

5. Repeat.

Glute Activation Warmups

Burpee

1. Stand straight up.

2. Bring both hands towards the floor, and once they're on the floor, extend both legs so they're straight behind you.

3. Jump or step your feet back to your hands.

4. Using your arms for momentum, jump up as high as you can while reaching your hands towards the ceiling.

6. Repeat until the set is complete!

Glute Activation Warmups

Clam Opener

1. Wrap the resistance band just over your knees

2. Lay on your leg side with your knees bent and your feet together.

3. Open your knees apart as widely as possible while squeezing the glute muscles in your right leg as tightly as possible.

4. Slowly allow the knee to come down so that they're together again on the floor, and repeat the movement.

Double Walk Out

1. Wrap the resistance bands around your calves or ankles.

2. Get into a squat position with your knees slightly bent and your feet shoulder-width apart.

3. Staying low in squat position, take a step to the right while maintaining the low squat position.

4. Step back to the original position, starting with your left leg.

5. Repeat.

*The double side step is the same movement, except you take two steps to the side and then return.

Glute Activation Warmups

Fire Hydrant

1. Wrap a resistance band around your thighs just above your knees.
2. Get into a Table-Top position with your knees and hands on the floor.
3. Keeping your knee bent, raise one leg laterally off the floor.
4. Repeat this until the set is complete.

*Can do this with or without the resistance band.

Glute Bridge w/Band Flutter

1. Lift your hips off the ground while keeping your toes pointed forward.

2. Open and close your knees together. When closing your knees, leave some tension in the band (don't close your legs all the way so the band doesn't get loose).

3. Try to keep your hips as centered as possible without dipping from side to side. Don't let your hips drop.

Note: Try and keep your hips as high as possible while doing this move.

Glute Activation Warmups

Glute Bridge w/Leg Extension

1. Lift your hips off the ground while keeping your toes pointed forward.

2. From here extend one leg while squeezing your glutes. If you alternate legs, make sure to keep your glutes squeezed.

3. Try to keep your hips as centered as possible without dipping from side to side. Don't let your hips drop.

Note: Try and keep your hips as high as possible while doing this move. Lateral Leg Raise w/ Flexed Foot.

Glute Activation Warmups

Lateral Leg Raise w/Foot Flexed

1. Lay on your side with your head resting in your hand.

2. From here, lift your leg up while keeping your foot flexed.

3. When returning your foot to the starting position, make sure to leave tension in the band (don't come low enough with your leg that the band becomes loose).

4. Repeat the movement while making sure your foot stays flexed.

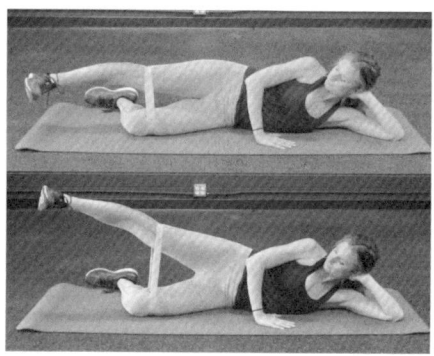

Lateral Leg Raise w/ Toes Pointing Down

1. Lay on your side with your head resting in your hand.

2. From here, lift your leg up while keeping your foot and toes pointed downwards.

3. When returning your foot to the starting position, make sure to leave tension in the band (don't come low enough with your leg that the band becomes loose).

4. Repeat the movement while making sure your foot stays pointed downwards.

Glute Activation Warmups

Lateral Lunge

1. Stand with your feet together.

2. Step out on one side into a lateral lunge, keeping your other foot straight.

3. Drop your butt as low as you can as if you're sitting in a chair, making sure your knees don't go past your toes in front of you.

4. From here, step back to center.

5. Repeat for duration of the set.

Glute Activation Warmups

Plank Knee Tuck

1. Get in a plank position with your hands on the floor, arms shoulder with apart and your body in a straight line.

2. From this position, bring your knee from your right leg under your body and over to your left elbow.

3. Return to plank position.

4. Alternate legs and repeat for the duration of the set.

Glute Activation Warmups

Running Man

1. Wrap the resistance band around your calves or ankles.

2. Get into an athletic position with your feet shoulder-width apart, knees slightly bent and your hips dropped.

3. Move your right foot backwards while staying slightly bent, and bring it back to the original position.

4. Repeat this quickly, but feel the glute contraction every time you complete the movement.

Glute Activation Warmups

Tabletop w/ Diagonal Kick

1. Get into a tabletop position with your hands and knees on the floor, and your back comfortably straight.

2. Raise one leg and straighten it.

3. As you straighten the leg, in one motion, move your straight leg behind the butt cheek on the other leg (the leg that is still on the floor).

4. Return to the original position and repeat.

Tabletop w/ Donkey Kick

1. Get into a tabletop position with your hands and knees on the floor and your back comfortably straight.

2. Raise one leg and straighten it out directly behind you while raising it as high as you possibly can. Make sure to feel the contraction in your glute muscles.

3. Allow the leg to slowly return to the original position and repeat.

4-3-2-1 Leg and Cardio Exercises

180 Jump Twist to Floor Tap

1. Get into a squat position, and then jump up and turn 180 degrees in the opposite direction.

2. As you land on the opposite side, touch the floor all in one motion with your right arm.

3. Jump back in the other direction and touch the floor with your left arm.

4. Repeat the movement until the set is complete.

Note: You can swing your arms to propel yourself back and forth.

3-Point Lunge

1. Starting with your feet together and your abs pulled in, step into a lateral lunge, making sure your stabilizing foot is straight. Step back to center.

2. Using the same leg, do a reverse lunge, and then step back to center.

3. With the same leg, do a curtsy lunge, and then repeat the entire movement.

4-3-2-1 Leg and Cardio Exercises

Bulgarian Lunge

1. Place one foot behind you on a platform.

2. While your foot is on the platform, bend your other foot into a 90% lunge.

3. Push up from the lunge by driving through your front heel to return to the original position.

4. Repeat.

Boxing Jab

1. Standing with the knees slightly bent, hold a light dumbbell in each hand.

2. Pivot your feet to one side and jab.

3. Come back to center, and then pivot your feet to the other side and jab with your other hand.

4. Repeat the movement while continuously alternating.

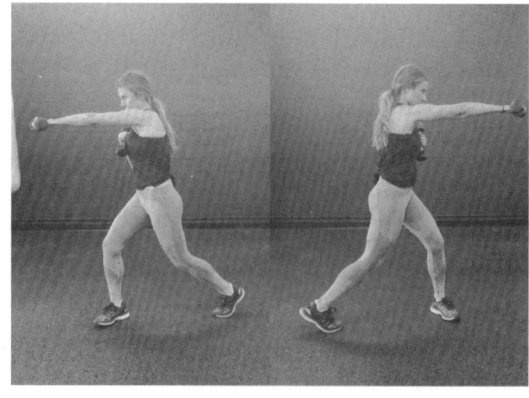

4-3-2-1 Leg and Cardio Exercises

Fast Feet

1. Start with your feet shoulder-width apart and your knees slightly bent.

2. Push through the balls of your feet an run in place, switching your feet as quickly as possible.

3. Stay low throughout the movement and move your arms as you do the running motion. Keep your spine neutral and your core tight!

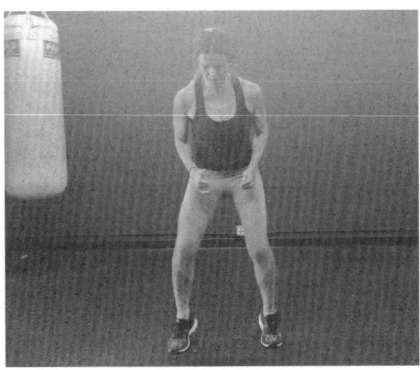

The Heisman

1. Jump or step onto your right foot and pull your left knee up towards your right shoulder as you jump.

2. Then jump onto your left foot while bringing your right knee up towards your left shoulder.

3. Repeat the movement until the set is complete.

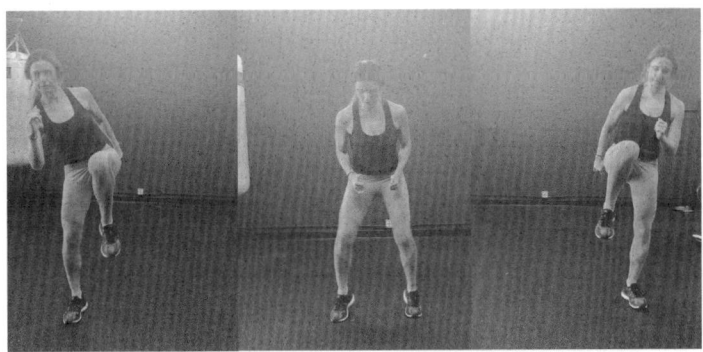

4-3-2-1 Leg and Cardio Exercises

High Knee

1. Stand straight up with your feet shoulder-width apart.

2. Run in place while raising your knees as high as possible as you alternate legs.

3. Repeat until the set is complete.

In and Out Jack

1. Stand straight up with your feet shoulder-width apart and holding dumbbells.

2. Jump into a wide squat position and touch the floor (or close to the floor) with one arm extended towards the floor.

3. Jump your feet back together in a straight, standing position.

4. Jump immediately back into a wide squat position and touch the floor with opposite hand.

5. Keep alternating arms back and forth.

*Try to keep your chest lifted while you do this.

4-3-2-1 Leg and Cardio Exercises

Jump Lunge

1. Step forward into a lunge position.

2. From here, explode out of your lunge into a jump, straightening both legs.

3. As you land, lower yourself back into another lunge with your other foot in front.

4. Stay low the entire time!

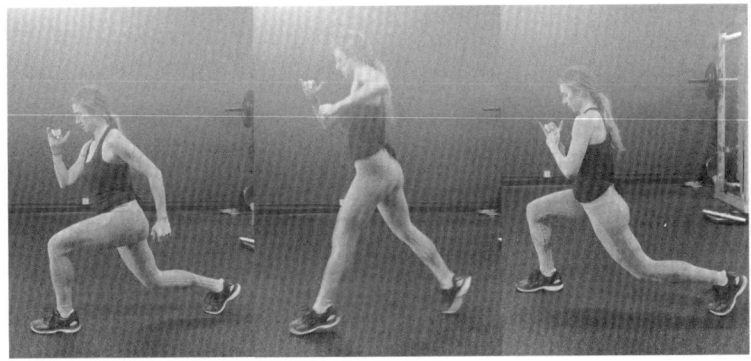

Jump Squat

1. In a squat position with feet shoulder-width apart and your weight in your heels, jump off the floor.

2. Jump, and land directly back in the squat position.

3. Repeat the movement until the set is complete.

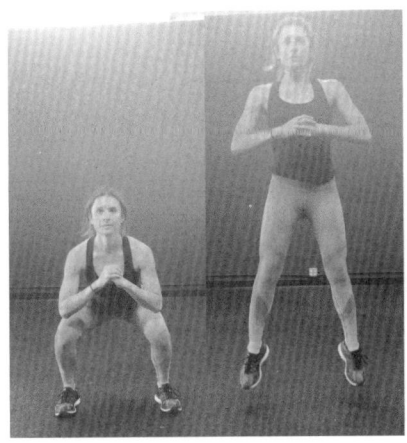

4-3-2-1 Leg and Cardio Exercises

Jump Twist

1. With your feet together, jump from side to side, while twisting your lower body.

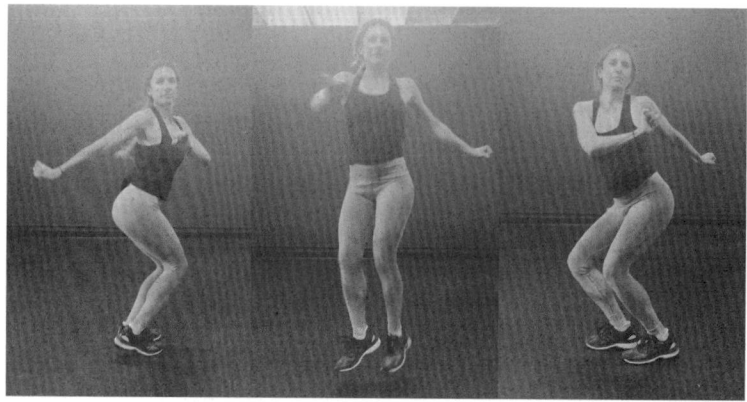

Lateral Lunge to Curtsy Lunge

1. Stand with your feet together, step out on one side into a lateral lunge, keeping your other foot straight. Drop your butt as low as you can as if you're sitting in a chair, making sure your knees don't go past your toes in front of you.

2. From here, step back to center, and with the same leg do a curtsy lunge take a big step back crossing it behind the stabilizer foot. Make sure to get your knee as close to the floor as possible!

3. Repeat for the duration of the set, and then switch sides.

4-3-2-1 Leg and Cardio Exercises

Lateral Lunge to Reverse Lunge

1. Stand with your feet together, step out on one side into a lateral lunge, keeping your other foot straight.

2. Drop your butt as low as you can as if you're sitting in a chair, making sure your knees don't go past your toes in front of you.

3. From here, step back to center, and with the same leg do a reverse lunge by taking a big step behind you. Make sure to get your knee as close to the floor as possible!

4. Repeat for the duration of the set, and then switch sides.

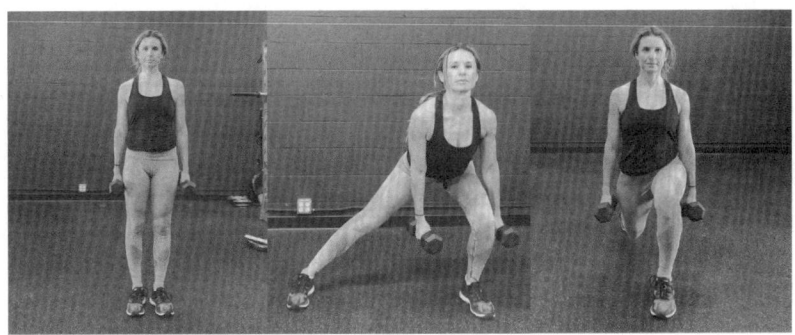

Lateral Lunge w/ Half 'X'

1. Place a dumbbell in your left hand and step out into a lateral lunge with your right leg.

2. Next, push out of your lunge by kicking off your right leg out and extending your left arm towards the ceiling.

3. Return to the starting position and repeat.

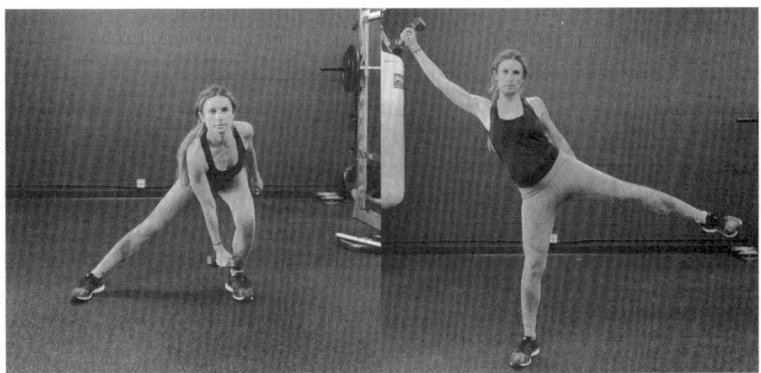

4-3-2-1 Leg and Cardio Exercises

Leap Forward in Squat, Burpee, & Shuffle Back

1. Get in a squat position with your feet shoulder width apart and your hips dropped towards the floor.

2. Leap forward as far as possible while staying low in squat position.

3. Quickly put your hands on the floor.

4. Extend your feet out behind you.

5. Pop your feet back in and stand up into your squat position.

6. Shuffle your feet back in very small steps, and repeat the movement.

Mountain Climber

1. Get in a push-up position with your hands directly underneath your shoulders.

2. From here, jump or step your right foot as close to your right hand as possible.

3. Then immediately jump or step your left foot as close to your left hand as possible while shifting your right leg back.

4. Keep alternating your legs as fast as you can.

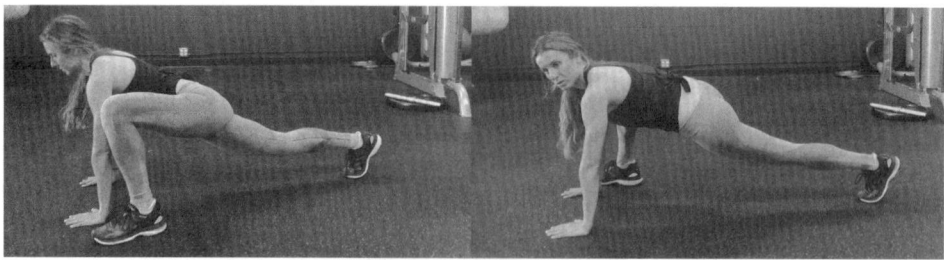

4-3-2-1 Leg and Cardio Exercises

Pendulum Jack

1. Hinge forward from your waist and place your hands on the floor in front of you.

2. Extend your right leg straight out to the side. Your left, supporting leg can be slightly bent.

3. From this position, quickly transfer your body-weight to the other leg.

4. Repeat the movement back and forth while keeping your hands on the ground until the set is complete.

Pendulum Lunge

1. Take a large step forward until your leg is making a 90 degree angle.

2. Take the same foot that lunged forward and do a reverse-lunge.

*To challenge your balance, try keeping your leg lifted from the front lunge to the reverse lunge rather than stepping back to center.

 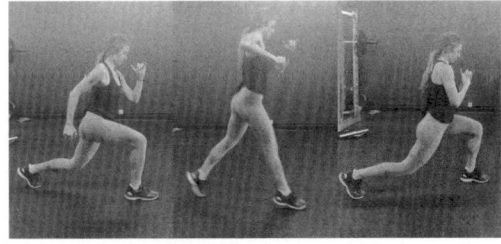

4-3-2-1 Leg and Cardio Exercises

Plank Jack

1. Get in a plank position with your hands on the floor, arms shoulder with apart and your body in a straight line.

2. From this position, jump your feet out and back in, as if you're doing a jumping jack.

*Bonus: Plank on your elbows instead of your hands to increase the difficulty of the exercise.

Plank Step Up, Alternating Arms

1. Get in push-up position, but rather than have your hands on the floor, put your elbows on the floor. Keep your body straight from your head to your feet.

2. Push off your right elbow onto your hand,

3. Then push off your left elbow onto your hand so now both of your hands are on the floor.

4. Then Drop from your right hand back onto your right elbow, and drop from your left hand to your left elbow.

5. Repeat the movement, starting with the left hand this time, until the set is complete.

*Keep your core tight throughout the exercise (and on all plank and leg exercises)!

*If this is difficult for you, keep your knees on the floor rather than your feet throughout the exercise.

4-3-2-1 Leg and Cardio Exercises

Plie Jump Squat

1. Point your toes outward so that they're facing the corners of the room, and then drop your hips into a Pile Squat position.

2. From here, jump up and then gently land directly back into the Pile Squat position.

3. Make sure your abs are pulled into your spine and your chest is lifted throughout the entire movement.

Bonus: touch your heels together when you are in the air.

Roundhouse Kick to Squat

1. Get into squat position.

2. Stand straight up, and as you stand up, shift your body to the right, and raise your left foot and kick out to the left.

3. As you're bringing your leg back to the floor, enter into the original squat position.

4. Repeat until the set is complete.

4-3-2-1 Leg and Cardio Exercises

Side Shuffle w/ Floor Tap

1. Starting in squat position, shuffle to the right three times and tap the floor.

2. Still staying low, shuffle three times to the left and tap the floor.

*Remember, stay in a low squat position throughout the whole set!

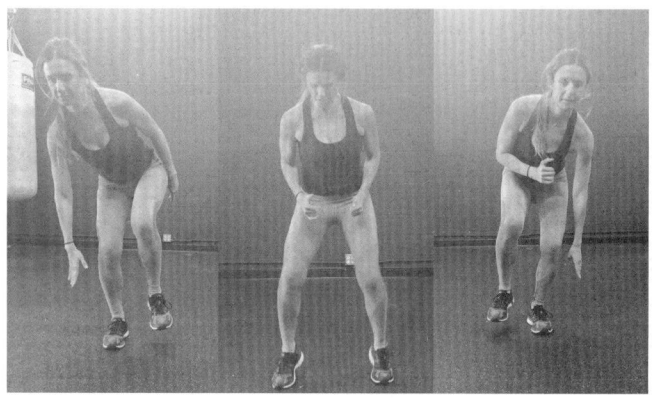

Side to Side Squat

1. Stand straight with your feet together, and holding dumbbells in each hand over your shoulder.

2. Take a step out to the right, press your hips back and squat with your weight in your heels.

3. Step your feet back together, and then squat to the left.

Bonus: Hold a weight with both hands for added resistance.

4-3-2-1 Leg and Cardio Exercises

Ski Mogul

1. Get into plank position with your feet together, jump both feet towards your right hand,

2. Then quickly jump your feet back to center position, and then jump your feet towards your left hand before jumping back to center position.

3. Keep repeating the alternating jumps until the set is complete.

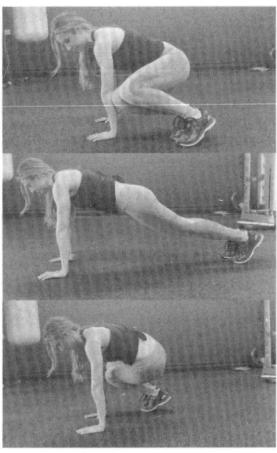

Speed Skater

1. Lean forward, jump to the right while bringing your left foot diagonally behind you, and your left arm in front of you.

2. Jump left, bringing your right arm in front of you and your right foot diagonally behind you.

3. Repeat this movement from side to side until the set is complete.

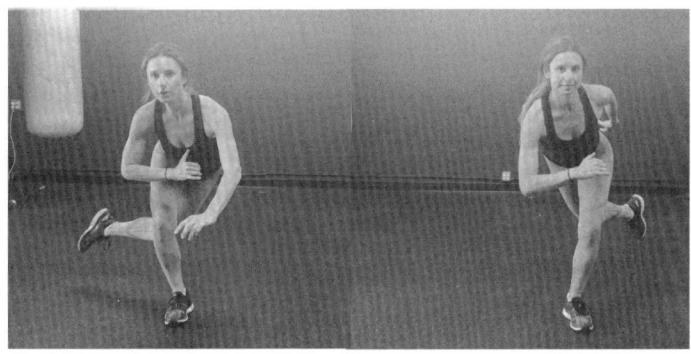

4-3-2-1 Leg and Cardio Exercises

Squat Jack

1. Stand in a squat position with your feet shoulder-width apart, knees bent and hips back towards the floor. Make sure the don't pass your toes.

2. From this position, jump and open your legs outwards for a bigger squat position, while staying low. Don't stand straight up in between.

3. Repeat until the set is complete.

Squat Thrust

1. Stand straight up.

2. Bring both hands towards the floor, and once they're on the floor, extend both legs so they're straight behind you.

3. Jump or step your feet back to your hands.

4. Stand straight up.

5. Repeat until the set is complete!

*Very similar to a burpee, just doesn't have the jump at the top.

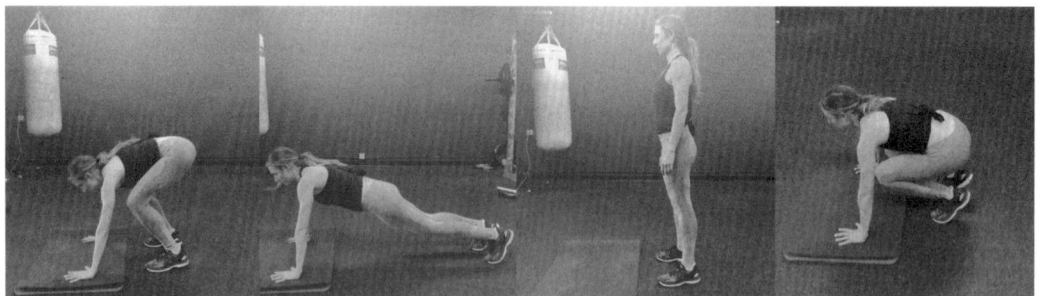

4-3-2-1 Leg and Cardio Exercises

Squat w/ Overhead Press

1. Holding a dumbbell on each shoulder, squat with your weight in your heels and knees aligned with your toes.

2. As you come back to starting standing position, press your dumbbells into the ceiling.

3. Return the weights to your shoulder and repeat the movement.

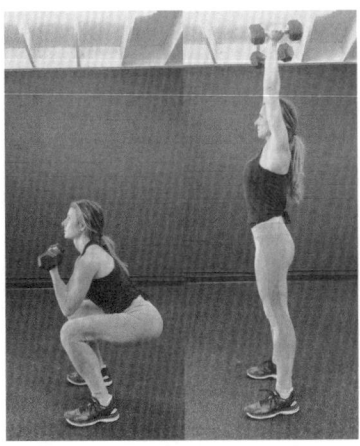

Vertical Leap

1. In a deep squat position with your weight in your heels and your booty as far back as possible, using your arms for momentum, jump up as high as you can while reaching your hands towards the ceiling.

2. Repeat this movement until the set is complete.

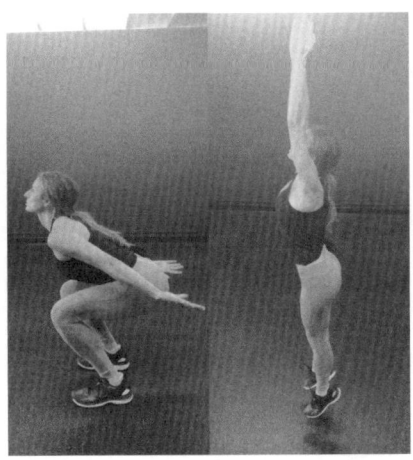

Weight Training Strength Exercises

Alternating Step Up

1. Hold a dumbbell in each hand, while keeping your core engaged and squeezing your glutes, step up onto a platform with your right foot (at a height that's comfortable for you,) step down, and then alternate sides.

2. Repeat.

Curtsy Lunge

1. Take a big diagonal step backwards with one leg, directly crossing it behind your other (stabilizing) and lower your leg until your knee is as close to the floor as possible.

Weight Training Strength Exercises

Deadlift

*Note: You can do this while holding dumbbells, or with a barbell

1. Holding dumbbells in each hand, keep your knees slightly bent and your back straight with your chest puffed outwards.

2. Hinging from your waist, bend down towards the floor as far as possible while keeping your back straight and your knees slightly bent.

3. At the climax of the movement (when you get as low as possible, hold for .5 - 1 seconds).

4. Using your legs and butt, straighten your knees until your body comes to a standing position.

5. Repeat the movement to complete the set.

*Because this exercise is more likely than others to lead to injury, please be very careful and make sure you understand proper form for Deadlifts before attempting to do the exercise.

Weight Training Strength Exercises

Elevated Plie Squat

1. Find two platforms, boxes, or benches that you can stand on with your feet separated so that there is space in between your legs and the platforms.

2. Get into a Plie Squat position by pointing your toes outwards towards the corners of the room, drop your hips and bend your knees slightly bent.

3. Holding a heavy weight in your hands, bend your knees and drop your hips towards the floor as low as possible for a DEEP squat.

4. Slowly come back up until your knees are only slightly bent and repeat the movement.

Weight Training Strength Exercises

Hip Thrust

1. Using a barbell or heavy dumbbell, use an amount of weight you're comfortable with.

2. Place your body under the barbell or put the dumbbell on the upper part of your thighs, and use a bench to support your back, neck, and head behind you.

3. Keep your feet on the floor, put your feet directly under your knees so that when you extend, you'll make a 90% angle.

4. Raise the barbell up from the floor primarily using your glute muscles.

5. Repeat the motion until the set is complete.

*It is VERY important to focus on contracting your glute muscles throughout this movement - make use of the mind-muscle connection! If you need to, slightly move your feet to see if you can get your glutes to fire.

*Make sure to maximize the full range of motion, going all the way up with your hips before coming back down slowly!

*If you're unsure what weight you're comfortable with, start off with something very light and see how it feels. Add to it until you find that comfortable but difficult weight level.

*You can use a pad or a towel under the bar for comfort

Weight Training Strength Exercises

Lateral Lunge w/ Knee to Elbow Rotation

1. Get into a lateral lunge position with your right leg bent close to a 90% angle and your left leg straight out.

2. As you push yourself out of the lunge, drive your left elbow to meet your right knee in the middle of your body. Make sure to engage your abs throughout the entire motion.

3. Repeat the movement.

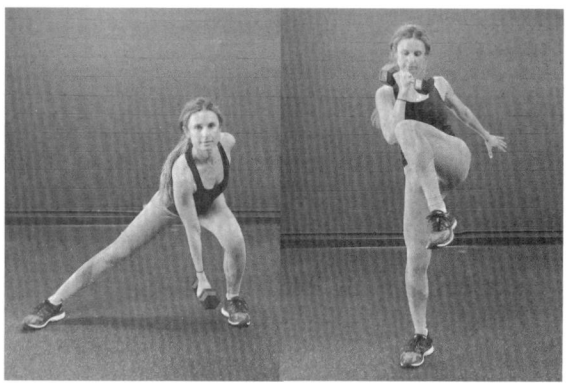

Plie Squat w/ Shoulder Windmill

1. Get into a deep Plie squat position with your hips dropped behind you, your knees slightly bent and feet shoulder-width apart. Feet should be pointed out towards the corners of the room.

2. Hold dumbbells in each hand with your palms facing away from your body.

3. As you squat down in this position, raise your arms up in a windmill motion, making a full-circle before your hands meet over your head.

4. Staying in this deep squat, lower your arms back down in the same windmill motion, and repeat the windmill motion until the set is complete.

Weight Training Strength Exercises

Single Leg Deadlift

1. Holding dumbbells in each hand, stand on one leg, keeping the standing leg slightly bent.

2. Hinge forward from your waist so your chest is almost parallel to the floor. Use your free leg for balance by straightening outwards behind you.

3. Lift your upper body back up to the original position using your hamstrings and glutes.

4. Repeat the movement.

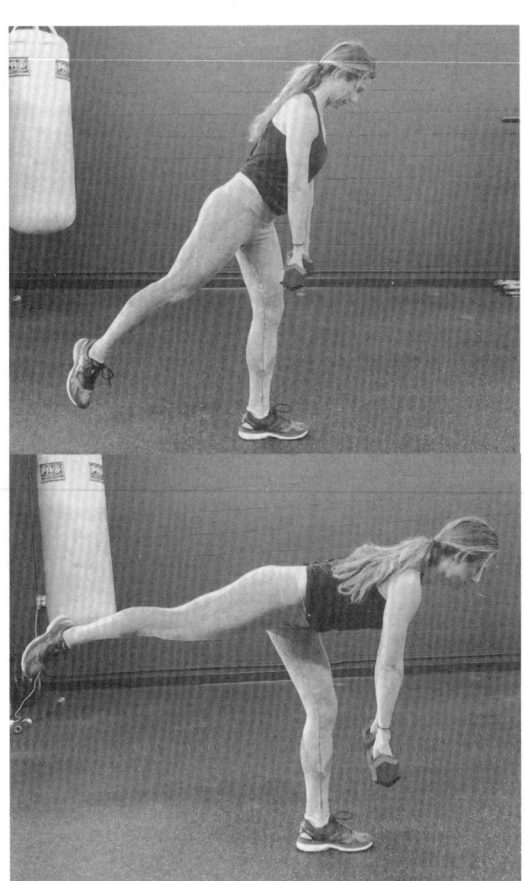

Weight Training Strength Exercises

Single Leg Glute Bridge

1. Lay on your back with your knees bent to a 90 degree angle. Place a heavy dumbbell on your lower stomach, and hold the dumbbell on both ends.

2. Using your glute muscles, lift your hips and pelvis as high off the floor as possible.

3. With a flexed foot, straighten and lift one leg towards the ceiling - this leg stays straight in the air.

4. Lower your body down so that it almost touches the floor while keeping one leg in the air.

5. Drive your hips up as high as possible again to repeat the movement.

Make sure not to let your hips dip.

Weight Training Strength Exercises

Squat

1. Set a bar (barbell or Smith Machine) on the height that best works for you.

2. Step under the bar and place the back of your shoulders (just under your neck) across the bar.

3. Hold on to the bar with both arms, palms facing forward.

4. Lift up to unlock the bar by pushing your legs up and raising your torso.

5. Twist your hands back to completely unlock the bar.

6. If you're not already, stand with your feet shoulder-width apart and your knees slightly bent for a squat position.

7. Bend your knees straight down as low as possible, and step straight back up while keeping your knees in line with your heels.

If you're unsure what weight you're comfortable with, start off with something very light and see how it feels. Add to it until you find that comfortable but difficult weight level.

Weight Training Strength Exercises

Woodchopper

1. Place a dumbbell on your left shoulder, holding it with both hands.

2. Step out into a forward lunge with your right leg, bending your right knee to a 90% angle.

3. As you lunge, rotate the dumbbell down and across your body, making a diagonal chopping motion.

4. As you push out of the lunge and stand back up, chop the dumbbell back up to your left shoulder.

Because this exercise can sound confusing, it's worth watching a video to make sure you understand how to complete the movement!

4-3-2-1 Waist Exercises

Leg Drop

1. Lie straight on the floor or on a flat bench. Place your hands underneath your lower back or butt and push your back into the floor.

2. Raise your legs together towards the ceiling, and then slowly lower them down so that they're hovering right above the floor.

3. Bring your legs right back up.

5. Repeat.

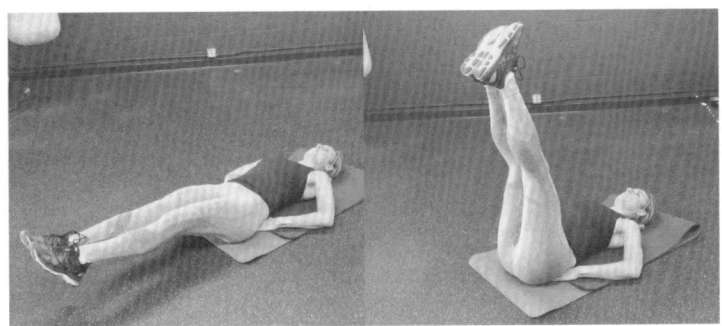

Russian Twist

1. Bend your knees and place your feet on the floor to make an imaginary 'V' shape with your body while holding yourself up. Lean your body back at a 45% angle and hold a dumbbell on both ends.

2. From here, rotate your body to one side and then shift to the other by twisting your torso.

You are never sitting straight up, you stay in the 45% angle and use your core to keep yourself stable.

Bonus: Keep your feet off the floor as you do this to work your lower abdominal muscles even more.

4-3-2-1 Waist Exercises

Side Plank w/ Elbow Twist

1. Get in plank position by placing your elbows and toes on the floor. Hold your body up off the floor in this position. With your free hand, place your fingertips behind your head.

2. From here, take your elbow and rotate towards the floor (try to touch your elbow to the floor).

3. Turn your torso back to the original position and repeat.

4. Repeat the movement until the set is complete before moving to the other side.

Side Plank w/ Torso Twist

1. Get in a side plank position by putting your left elbow on the floor, and lifting yourself off the floor with your left elbow (You can either stack your feet or stagger your feet. Stacking is more difficult).

2. Hold a dumbbell in your right hand and straighten your arm towards the ceiling.

3. While holding this position, rotate your torso and lower the hand with the weight under and through your torso.

3. Place it on the floor for one second, and then rotate your torso back to the original position and repeat.

4. While doing so keep your hips lifted off the floor the entire time.

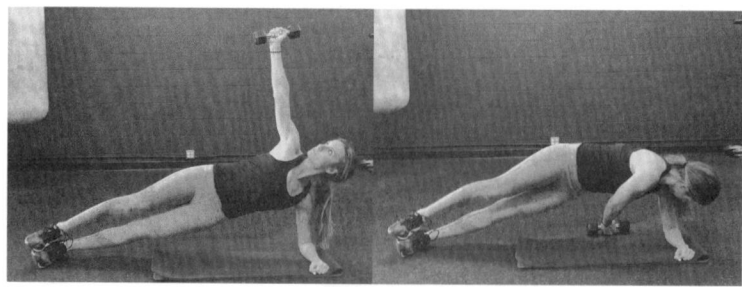

4-3-2-1 Waist Exercises

Side Triangle Crunch

1. Get in a side plank position by putting your left elbow on the floor, and lifting yourself off the floor with your left elbow (You can either stack your feet or stagger your feet. Stacking is more difficult).

2. Hold a dumbbell in your right hand and straighten your arm towards the ceiling.

3. While holding this position, lower your elbow and raise your knee so that they meet in the middle of your body.

4. While doing so keep your hips lifted off the floor the entire time.

Side V-Up

1. Lie on your left side, legs straight out and angled 30 degrees from your hips. Keep your left arm on the floor, your right arm behind your head.

2. Raise your legs from the floor while simultaneously bringing your torso up (primarily using the right side of your abdominal muscles) towards your legs.

3. Complete the same movement with the left side

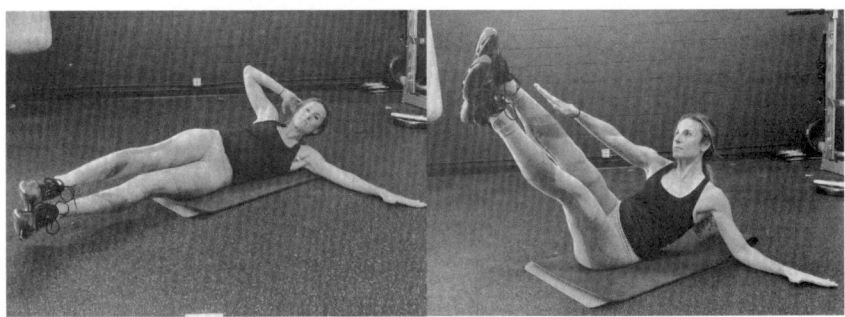

4-3-2-1 Waist Exercises

Spider-man Plank Crunch

1. Get in plank position by placing your elbows and toes on the floor Hold your body up off the floor in this position.

2. Bring your right knee on the outside of your body to your right elbow.

3. Straighten your right leg back to the floor.

4. Complete the same movement with your left leg, and keep alternating sides.

Standing Side Crunch

1. Stand with your feet a little more than hip-distance apart.

2. With a dumbbell in each hand, raise one dumbbell up and over your head - your arm should be straight.

3. From here, crunch to the side by lowering your arm while raising your knee so that your elbow and knee meet in the middle of your body. Bring your knee as far up to the side of your body as possible.

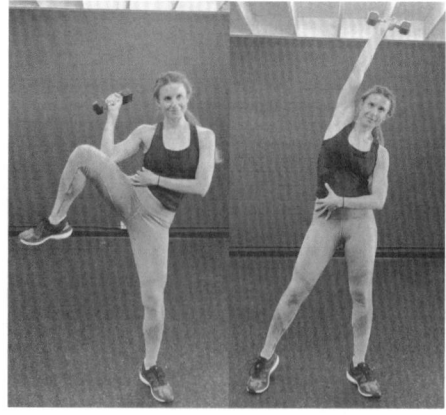

4-3-2-1 Waist Exercises

Starfish Crunch

1. Lie flat on the floor (on your backside)

2. Open your arms and legs wide to make a starfish shape

3. Bring your left leg straight up and simultaneously bring your right hand to meet your left leg in the middle of your body, for a complete body crunch.

4. Alternate sides.

5. Repeat until the set is complete!

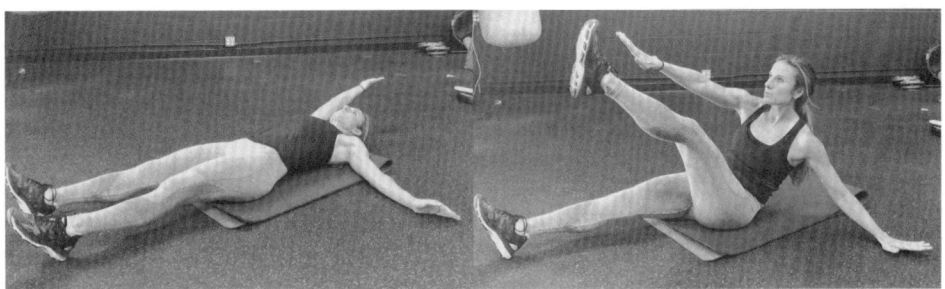

Tabletop w/ Elbow to Knee Crunch

1. Get in a tabletop position with your hands directly beneath your shoulders. Hold your body up off the floor in this position. Hold a light dumbbell in your right hand.

2. From this position extend your right arm out in front of you, and extend your left leg straight out behind you.

3. Next, crunch your abs by bringing your right elbow to meet your left knee in the middle of your body.

4. Extend them again and repeat.

5. Make sure to finish one side before switching hands and doing the other side.

4-3-2-1 Waist Exercises

Vertical Sit-Up w/ Elbow to Knee Touch

1. Lie on your back with one leg bent and the other leg extended off the ground. Your fingertips should be behind your head.

2. From this position, twisting from the waist, get your right elbow to meet your left knee in the middle of your body.

3. Straighten your body.

4. Simultaneously bring your left knee in while raising and twisting your torso and right elbow into your left knee.

5. Repeat the movement.

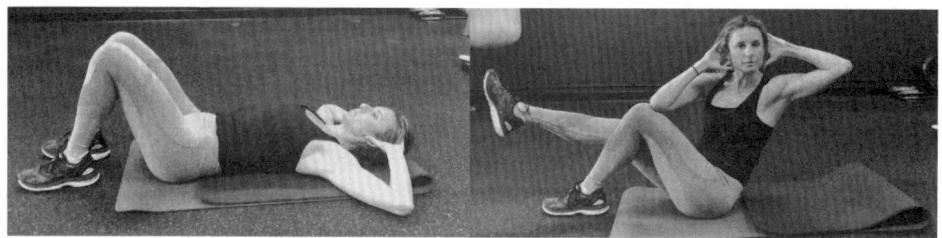

V-Up

1. Lie straight on your back with your legs together and your arms together straight above your head.

2. In one motion, raise your legs off the floor while keeping them straight. Also raise your torso and hands to meet your legs in the middle of your body.

3. Repeat!

Shoulder & Back Exercises

Bent Over Row

You can either use dumbbells or a barbell for this exercise

1. Hold dumbbells in each hand or take a barbell and allow it to hang in front of you.
2. Hinging forward from your waist, keep your knees slightly bent and keep your back straight.
3. Drive your elbows back while squeezing your shoulder blades together. Hold for 1 second, and go back to the starting position slowly.
4. Repeat the movement.

*If you have lower back problems, try to find an alternative for this exercise like a seated row.

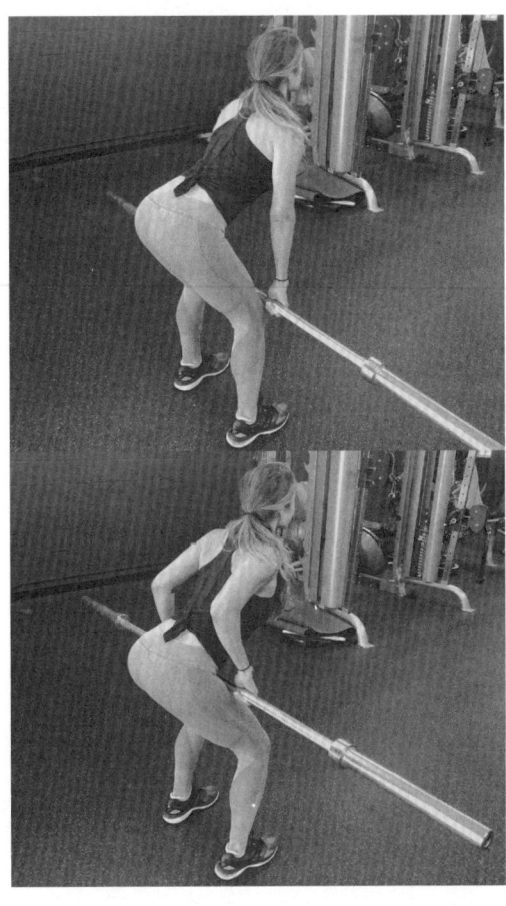

Shoulder & Back Exercises

Lateral Raise

*Can complete this exercise sitting down on a bench, or standing up. This is also combined with squats in our workouts.

1. Stand up straight with your feet shoulder width apart and have dumbbells by your side at arms length away. When performing this exercise your palms should be facing down.

2. Keep your abs pulled into your spine, your torso stationary and raise the dumbbells to your side with a slight bend at your elbow. Lift your arms until they are parallel to the floor (shoulder level) and pause for a second at the top.

3. Lower the dumbbells back down slowly and repeat.

Lat Pulldown

1. Grab a wide grip handle bar. Adjust the knee pad of the machine to fit your height to prevent your body from being raised while performing the movement.

2. Grasp the bar with an overhand grip and your palms facing forward. For a wide grip, your grip on the bar should be wider than shoulder width apart.

3. Keep your torso stationary and pull the bar down towards your upper chest. Squeeze your back muscles during the movement.

5. Slowly raise the bar in a controlled motion back to the starting position, with your arms are fully extended and lats fully stretched.

Shoulder & Back Exercises

Plank to Row

1. Holding a dumbbell in each hand, get into a push-up position with your hands directly beneath your shoulders. Keep your abs pulled into your spine.

2. Drive your elbow up towards the ceiling while keeping your arm as close to your ribcage as possible.

3. Lower the weight back to the ground and complete the same movement on the other side.

4. Keep alternating until the set is complete.

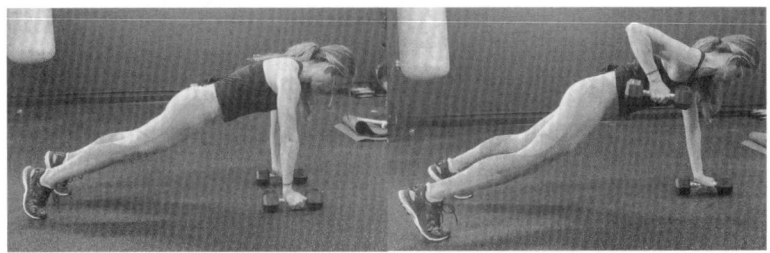

Reverse Dumbbell Fly

1. Grab a dumbbell in each hand.

2. Bend your knees slightly and hinging forward from your hips so that your upper body is leaning comfortably forward towards the floor.

3. Hold the dumbbells out together in front of your torso with your arms as straight as possible.

4. Pull the dumbbells out away from your body while keeping your arms almost fully extended, as if you were trying to squeeze your shoulder blades together.

5. Slowly return to the original position, still keeping your arms straight.

6. Repeat the movement until the set is complete!

Shoulder & Back Exercises

Shoulder Rope Pull

1. Stand with the rope in between your legs.

2. Keeping your arms straight (elbows *slightly* bent), pull the rope up from the floor to your shoulder height, hold for a count of two seconds, and slowly return to the starting position.

3. Repeat until the set is complete.

Straight Arm Rope Pull or Bar Pull

The movement is the same whether you're using a rope or a bar!

1. Find a pulldown machine and attach a wide bar from at your shoulder level on the pulley. Grab the bar with an overhand grip (palms facing down), and make sure your grip is wider than your shoulder-width.

2. Take a couple steps back and keep your feet shoulder-width apart. Slightly hinge at the waist so your torso is leaning forward. Keep your arms fully extend, so that' it's parallel with the ground, and have a slight bend at the elbows.

3. Pull the bar down while keeping the arms straight. Continue pulling down until your hands are beside your thighs; you should feel a contraction in your lats.

4. Repeat the movement.

Shoulder & Back Exercises

Arnold Press

*Can complete this exercise sitting down on a bench, or standing up. This is also combined with squats in our workouts.

1. Hold a dumbbell in each hand, raise your arms so that your palms are facing your face with your elbows close together.

3. Push the dumbbells up over your head while simultaneously twisting your hands so when your hands are straight over your head, your palms are facing outwards.

4. Bend your arms while twisting your hands so that you go back to the original position.

5. Repeat the movement!

Shoulder & Back Exercises

Cable Row w/Squat

Caution: Avoid swinging your torso back and forth as you can cause a lower back injury.

You can use a rope, two handles, or a V-bar to complete this exercise.

1. Attach a rope to a low pulley on a cable.

2. Grab the rope, and sit back in a squat position as close to 90 degrees as possible. Make sure you're far back enough that you have full range of motion with your arms.

3. Pull the rope as far back as possible by driving your elbows directly behind you. Squeeze your shoulder blades together, hold for 1 second, and then return to the starting position.

4. Repeat the movement until the set is complete.

Stretches

Butterfly Stretch

1. Sitting in an upright position with your back straight, and your chest lifted.

2. Put the soles of your feet together, and push down on your knees gently to get a deep stretch in your groin and inner thighs.

Crossbody Hangover

1. Cross one foot over the other, and hinging from your waist, hang your upper body over your lower body and try to touch the floor with your arms. Feel the stretch in your hamstrings, and try to lengthen your spine.

2. Switch feet and continue the stretch.

Stretches

Glute Stretch

1. Lying on your back, place one leg over the other and pull your leg towards your chest.

Hamstring Stretch

1. Lying on your back with one leg fully extended, bring the other leg up towards your chest while trying to keep your leg as straight as you can.

2. From here, flex and point your toes towards the ceiling. Switch legs and repeat.

Stretches

Lat Stretch

1. Inch your fingers up the wall until you feel a stretch on the side of your body in your lats.

Pigeon Stretch

1. Sit with your right knee bent in front of you, and your left leg extended behind you. Pull your right heel in towards your left hip.

2. Lean forward until you feel a deep stretch in your glutes and hips.

Stretches

Runner's Stretch

1. Lunge forward with one leg at a 90 degree angle while your other foot remains straight behind you with the bottom of your foot facing the ceiling.

2. Gently press through your hips. Lift your opposite arm up towards the ceiling.

3. If you're flexible enough, try lifting your foot and grabbing your toes.